RISK AND LUCK IN MEDICAL ETHICS

To Anders and Pip, two bits of outcome luck.

RISK AND LUCK IN MEDICAL ETHICS

Donna Dickenson

polity

Copyright © Donna Dickenson 2003

The right of Donna Dickenson to be identified as author of this work has been asserted in accordance with the Copyright, Designs and Patents Act 1988.

First published in 2003 by Polity Press in association with Blackwell Publishers Ltd, a Blackwell Publishing Company.

Editorial office:
Polity Press
65 Bridge Street
Cambridge CB2 1UR, UK

Marketing and production:
Blackwell Publishers Ltd
108 Cowley Road
Oxford OX4 1JF, UK

Published in the USA by
Blackwell Publishers Inc.
350 Main Street
Malden MA 02148, USA

A catalogue record for this book is available from the British Library.

Library of Congress Cataloging-in-Publication Data

Dickenson, Donna.
  Risk and luck in medical ethics / Donna Dickenson.
    p. cm.
Includes bibliographical references and index.
  ISBN 0–7456–2145–7 (alk. paper) — ISBN 0–7456–2146–5 (pbk.: alk. paper)

1. Medical ethics. 2. Risk. 3. Fortune. 4. Uncertainty. I. Title.
R725.5 .D533 2002
174'.2—dc21   2002003389

Typeset in 10.5 on 12pt Sabon
by Kolam Information Services Pvt. Ltd., Pondicherry, India.
Printed in Great Britain by MPG Books Ltd, Bodmin, Cornwall
This book is printed on acid-free paper.

Contents

Preface

In formal terms, *Risk and Luck in Medical Ethics* is the second edition of my 1991 book *Moral Luck in Medical Ethics and Practical Politics*. In other senses – not least in that many of the chapters are entirely new, and others greatly rewritten – it is something more than a second edition. The core of my argument has not changed, but the applications have broadened in one sense and narrowed in another. I have decided to concentrate more exclusively on medical ethics, although not to the exclusion of a new topic, global ethics, which I consider in chapter 10. For reasons that should become somewhat intelligible to the reader in chapter 2, and clearer in chapter 10, the operations of luck can be argued to undermine the possibility of reaching any sort of agreement on what ethics offers and demands, or the formulation of any set of common values. Luckily – if the pun can be excused – the situation is not so dire as that. Using a model drawn from feminist theory, I conclude that the paradox of moral luck does not abolish the possibility of a common core set of values, or indeed the possibility of there being such a thing as 'ethics'; rather, it concentrates the mind wonderfully on what ethics can sensibly hope to achieve.

The areas to which I extend medical ethics are more numerous and, I think, more challenging than those in the first edition, which were limited to informed consent and the allocation of scarce medical resources. I now include chapters on psychiatric ethics (where risk enters into assessments of dangerousness, for example); reproductive ethics (where new reproductive technologies such as therapeutic cloning and contract motherhood raise the question of what risks women can be asked to bear); genetics (where the possibility that our behaviour is genetically determined raises questions about purposiveness in action and luck in character); and death and dying (where there is a new risk that technology may extend the semblance of life when the conditions for a meaningful life have gone). The chapters on informed consent and resource allocation remain, as does the essential argument in each: in the first case, that the purpose of informed consent is to transfer responsibility for ill-luck in outcomes from doctor to patient; in the second, that randomized allocation mechanisms such as lotteries and waiting lists 'draw luck's fire' and are to be preferred over supposedly more objective clinical measures. Particularly in the case of resource allocation, the prevailing trend ten years after the first book is in the opposite direction, towards evidence-based medicine as the main tool for policy decisions about what treatments to fund, and I have updated the chapter to demonstrate some of the pitfalls of relying solely on allocation on that basis as an attempt to avoid the depredations of luck and chance.

These are the six practical chapters of the book, chapters 4 through 9; in addition to the final chapter on global ethics, there are three initial theoretical chapters which both set the stage and provide what I hope is a properly analytical argument about how and why luck can be said to be inimical to moral systems. Luck is more hostile to ethical consequentialism than to Kantianism, I argue, although at first things look to be the other way round. In this edition I also consider the position of luck in virtue ethics, which has come into its own since I first wrote.

In the past decade notions about risk and luck have simultaneously come to the fore and been systematically erased from policy-making. The concept of the 'risk society' has entered academic parlance (Ulrich Beck, *Risk Society: Towards a New Modernity*), but in public policy risk has been systematically transferred from governments to individuals. We are now more and more responsible for our own pension provision, health care insurance, and other forms of 'thinking ahead', with governments seeking to reduce the role of the state when things go wrong. On the other hand, the concepts of risk and significant harm have entered the statute books in the UK with the Children Act 1989 and the Mental Health (Patients in the Community) Act 1995, as well as in the debate over amending the Mental Health Act 1983. Frequently, however, governments have oversimplified the operations of risk, or sought to avoid them altogether. Here I have in mind the 'three strikes and you're out' model of criminal justice which holds increasing sway in both the USA and the UK: rather than forming a probabilistic assessment of the likelihood of a further crime being committed by someone who has offended three times, even on minor charges, this model shuts down judgements of risk altogether, by effectively saying that the likelihood is 100 per cent. Perhaps it is not surprising that, when we feel increasingly vulnerable to the operations of risk and luck, we should seek to deny them. (And we are more likely to feel that nothing is secure after the murders of 11 September 2001.) But the argument in this book is that only by recognizing risk and luck openly, and by explicitly incorporating them into decision-making in medical ethics and elsewhere, can we transcend ill-luck in outcomes and other forms of 'moral luck'.

Finally, an apology to those readers who might have been expecting me to produce a further full-scale work on property following my 1997 book *Property, Women and Politics*. I have been continuing to develop my work on property in the body and in reproductive labour, with most of my research appearing in articles and book chapters so far (see bibliography). A recent Wellcome Trust-funded initiative on commodification of pregnancy-related tissue has also helped me to develop my thought and should soon see further publications. In this book, chapter 7, on risk in reproductive ethics, does contain substantial further development of the 1997 volume's position on contract motherhood.

I would like to express my gratitude to all those who have helped me to develop case material and concepts used in this book: the Academic Department of Psychiatry at the Warneford Hospital, Oxford; the Riverside Mental Health Trust clinical ethics committee, London; St Mary's Hospital clinical ethics committee, London; my former colleagues at Imperial College School of Medicine, London; my current colleagues at the Centre for the Study of Global Ethics, University of Birmingham, particularly Helen Harris for her calm and patience in preparing the final manuscript; Thomas Murray, Dan Callahan, Angela Wasunna and other staff of the Hastings Center, USA; Dr Jim Howe of Airedale NHS Trust, whom I had the good fortune to interview for an Open University programme on the case of Tony Bland, who was his patient; Alan Ryan, warden of New College, Oxford, and Professor Tom Sorrell of the University of Essex, who supervised the doctoral dissertation on which the first edition of this book was based; David Lamb, series editor for the first edition; Noam Zohar, who has consistently encouraged my work on moral luck from the time the first book appeared in print; members of the Feminist Approaches to Bioethics group, particularly Rosemarie Tong (whose ideas were crucial to chapter 10) and Mary Mahowald (of whom the same can be said for chapter 9); partners and participants in my three European projects, EBEPE (European Biomedical Ethics Practitioner Education), TEMPE (Teaching Ethics: Materials for Practitioner Education) and Evibase (Ethical issues in evidence-based medicine); and finally David Held and Gill Motley at Polity, for their unflagging enthusiasm about the second edition despite the very flagging progress I frequently made with it.

Very few of these people agree with all my arguments about risk and luck, of course, and some radically disagree. This is the stuff of academic debate, but I have been very fortunate in that the debate has not been merely academic. It is a continuing source of pleasure and amazement to me to see how seriously ethics is taken by clinicians in their teaching, on research and clinical ethics committees, and in their everyday rounds. While some academics, such as Bernard Williams or the post-modern thinkers, seem to me all too willing to give up on ethics as an enterprise, I find that those 'at the coalface' almost inevitably want to talk and know more about ethics. I hope that this book may help them: it is certainly intended to be relevant and intelligible to clinicians. Readers without some background in philosophy may find the first three chapters and the final chapter more difficult than those with such training, but the moral philosophy in those chapters is not highly technical.

Grateful acknowledgement is also made to Oxford University Press for permission to reproduce (in chapters 8 and 9) material from case studies in Donna Dickenson and K. W. M. Fulford, *In Two Minds: case studies in psychiatric ethics* (2001).

Donna Dickenson
Beckley, Oxford

1

Ethics versus Luck?

The myriad forms of luck

Is 'moral' incompatible with luck? The attempt to shore up the ethically right against the tidal waves of ill-chance is often thought central to ethical thought. If it fails, is ethics as a whole somehow at risk? Ethics is commonly assumed to be the one realm in which luck does not intrude. 'While one can be lucky in one's business, in one's married life, and in one's health, one cannot, so it is commonly assumed, be subject to luck as far as one's moral worth is concerned.'[1]

The imperviousness of ethics to luck is central to the 'appeal' of ethics. If ethics is not impervious to luck, the notion of the moral enterprise as a universal good suffers doubly. First, justice as equality is threatened: it is not open to some – those tainted by the particular kinds of ill-luck that I shall come to – to be as moral as those who are not so affected. Secondly, justice as desert is infringed: 'if morality depends on luck, then at least sometimes people are judged morally for things that are beyond their control.'[2]

Typically we maintain two incompatible standards towards right actions and good character, and the tension between these polarities creates the paradox of moral luck. In practice we regard actions as right or wrong, and moral character as good or bad, partly according to what happens as a result of the agent's decision. That is, we make responsibility hinge to some extent on things outside the agent's control. Yet at the same time we think that people should not be held responsible for matters beyond their control.

This tension underpins Kant's famous assertion that only the good will is securely good, and that its goodness is impervious to ill-luck in how things actually turn out.

Even if it should happen that by a particularly unfortunate fate or by the niggardly provision of a stepmotherly nature, this will should be wholly lacking in power to accomplish its purpose, if even the greatest effort should not avail it to achieve anything of its end, and if there remained only the good will (not as a mere wish, but as the summoning of all the means in our power), it would sparkle like a jewel in its own right, as something that had full worth in itself.[3]

But is moral luck only a problem for a Kantian? Perhaps only one particular school of ethics is vulnerable to moral luck arguments, but ethics as a whole is not. That would be a reassuring conclusion for clinicians and philosophers alike. However, there is a increasing consensus that the moral luck problem is larger than that. Martha Nussbaum, for example, has claimed that not only Kant but also Plato was motivated by a concern to minimize the effects of chance on moral character and the rightness of ethical choices.[4] Although ethical consequentialism, including utilitarianism, appears not to have a problem with moral luck, it actually does, as I shall argue in chapter 3. Indeed, Bernard Williams, who originated the term 'moral luck', has always maintained that moral luck is a problem for ethics in general, not merely for Kantian ethics in particular:

> [Non-Kantians] may be disposed to think, so far as morality is concerned, that all that is in question is the pure Kantian conception, and that conception merely represents an obsessional exaggeration. But it is not merely that, nor is the Kantian attempt to escape luck an arbitrary enterprise. The attempt is so intimate to our notion of morality, in fact, that its failure may rather make us consider whether we should not give up that notion altogether.[5]

If the paradox of moral luck is a genuine paradox, and if its applicability is really so vast, then the scope of our examination needs to be narrowed. In this book I want to examine whether the concepts of luck and risk can cast any light on problems in medical ethics, and, conversely, whether grounding the concepts of luck and risk in practical ethics might help up to better understand and perhaps resolve the paradox. The moral luck debate, begun by Bernard Williams and Thomas Nagel in 1976,[6] has become reasonably familiar to many philosophers, but is still comparatively little known in medical ethics proper.[7] This is unfortunate, since the concept of moral luck can offer a good deal of help to clinical ethicists, health care professionals and students, managers and others involved in making decisions in medical ethics. The basic question to ask is simple: what happens if things go wrong?

In the first three chapters, I erect the theoretical framework for what I hope will actually be a more sophisticated discussion than might be suggested by the basic question of what happens when things beyond an agent's control do go wrong. I begin in this chapter with a systematic exposition of the moral luck debate between Williams and Nagel, considering also the ramifications of the debate in further articles on the same subject by other writers.[8] I explore Williams's own further reflections on the significant debate which he set in train.[9] Whether the paradox is genuine, and, if it is a true paradox, the range of its effects on ethics, are also considered.

The second chapter begins by examining moral luck and virtue ethics. The moral luck debate was extended by Martha Nussbaum in *The Fragility of Goodness*, which concluded that only an Aristotelian, virtue-centred approach can overcome the paradox. The current popularity of virtue ethics in medicine[10] perhaps rests on its concern with what sort of doctor it is good to be, rather than what action is prescribed in disconnected individual decisions. This chapter will counter the accepted wisdom by arguing that a classical, virtue-centred approach does not in fact get round the problem of risk and luck in medical decision-making. Using Nussbaum's critique of Kant as a bridge, I also analyse the deontological, Kantian sources of the claim that ethics cannot allow itself to be undermined by chance. Nussbaum's rather conventional interpretation of Kant presents him as particularly prone to the moral luck paradox, in what she views as an attempt to create a risk-free ethics in which there remains only the good will. I shall argue instead that Kant wants conscience to have an impact on the world, and that a Kantian approach to dilemmas in the medical world, such as informed consent, actually offers a promising way forward, by limiting what it is that we are actually responsible for but interpreting that responsibility strictly.

In chapter 3 I turn from virtue ethics and deontology to ethical consequentialism, and particularly to utilitarianism. In contrast to deontology, utilitarianism makes the moral agent responsible for too much, and is particularly vulnerable to the paradox of moral luck. This is true even if the agent is responsible not for actual but for potential consequences. Three important concepts associated with moral luck are explored in this chapter: risk, probability and rationality. Chapters 2 and 3 are intended for the reader with philosophical interests, although they do not require any substantial philosophical background.

The reader whose interests are primarily clinical may prefer to press on to the applied chapters and to the conclusion in chapter 10. However, it might be worth a brief stopover at the section on remorse and regret at the end of chapter 3.

The applied, practical chapters of the book, chapters 4 through 9, concern, respectively:

- risk and luck in informed consent to treatment
- moral luck in decisions about withholding life-sustaining treatment
- moral luck in the allocation of scarce medical resources
- risk and luck in reproductive ethics, with particular focus on contract motherhood ('surrogacy'), and in cloning
- risk in psychiatry
- genetics and luck in character.

In several of these chapters, particularly those on allocation of resources, reproductive ethics and research ethics, I deliberately take a 'global' focus. I do not confine resource allocation to decisions within one jurisdiction; I consider the possible exploitation of third-world women as egg donors in stem cell technologies; and I ask questions about what risks it is permissible for first-world researchers to impose on third-world populations. The last chapter, chapter 10, considers the wider ramifications for global ethics of value pluralism, which Williams insists is the logical corollary of accepting that luck does fatally undermine ethics. In a final synthesis, I argue that radical value pluralism and its associated strands in global ethics can be avoided, and that we can look to similar debates in feminist theory about difference and identity to help us find a way out of the dilemma.

A preliminary typology of luck

In this first chapter I summarize the Williams–Nagel debate, and ask whether the moral luck paradox is genuine. Before I begin, however, I need to distinguish among various types of luck. The moral luck paradox has generally been construed as being primarily about *luck in outcomes or consequences*, with the question of what kinds of consequences we are responsible for. Within outcome luck, one might further distinguish (as does Ronald Dworkin) between *option luck* and *'brute' luck*. As Dworkin puts it:

Option luck is a matter of how deliberate and calculated gambles turn out – whether someone gains or loses through accepting an isolated risk he or she should have anticipated and might have declined. Brute luck is a matter of how risks fall out that are not in that sense deliberate gambles. If I buy a stock on the exchange that rises, then my option luck is good. If I am hit by a falling meteorite whose course could not have been predicted, then my bad luck is brute (even though I could have moved just before it struck if I had any reason to know where it would strike).[11]

The moral language of 'should' ('should have anticipated and might have declined') can apply only to option luck, which involves *choice* as opposed to mere *chance* (or, more properly, involves choice as well as chance). Put another way, I am responsible for the decisions which are involved in option luck, even though I am not solely responsible for the consequences. If my stock rises, I might congratulate myself on my financial acumen; if it falls, I might blame myself for choosing badly, for not getting out of a bear market sooner, or for indulging in the high-flown gambling which is the stock market in the first place. The extent to which I am responsible is precisely what we want to determine, and what gives rise to the paradox of moral luck. But although I might rue the moment I unwittingly stood in the path of the meteorite (assuming I somehow survive), it would be unreasonable of me to blame myself for my brute ill-luck. Later I will introduce a somewhat similar distinction made by Bernard Williams between regret and remorse, and a parallel distinction which he draws between luck intrinsic to the agent's 'project' and luck extrinsic to it.

Ethical issues are not present in the second subcategory of outcome luck – brute luck – but neither are they confined to outcome luck alone. Outcome luck focuses our intention on results, but we must also look to luck in causal factors. If I give £10 to Oxfam as an expression of my belief that it is ethically desirable to help feed the hungry, I do not regard my decision as having been proved unethical by a flash flood which stops the supplies that I have donated from getting through.[12] However, I am of course lucky to have £10 to give, so that my generosity is somehow slightly less than mine alone: it is partly also a matter of my good fortune in living in a comparatively wealthy country and being in work. (Of course, some people live in a first-world country, hold paid employment, and do not contribute to charity, so my generosity is partly my own.) This can be seen as a form of *circumstantial luck*, or *luck in antecedent circumstances*, to use Thomas Nagel's terminology.[13] The sixth chapter of this book, on fair distribution of scarce medical resources, will concern luck in antecedent circumstances as well as outcome luck.

I am also lucky to live under a watered-down version of Christianity which does not demand that I sell all I have and give my goods to the poor. I can be accounted generous only because the moral standards set by my society are actually rather lax in the matter of financial altruism, so that in another sense of 'luck' I am lucky to live in this society. This is what Nagel calls *luck in the problems which have to be faced.*[14] Still using the same example, these days I may not necessarily be praised for my contribution to Oxfam if my motivation is naively to 'feed the poor'. The debate has got more difficult than that: to the extent that 'humanitarian' assistance reinforces patronizing images of third-world dependency, or only serves the 'bureaucracy of the aid system',[15] then perhaps my donation is not so praiseworthy after all. Increasing awareness of 'colonialist' patterns in development work over the past ten to twenty years has increased the problems which have to be faced in deciding whether and how to give support to countries of the South. Perhaps I am actually unlucky in that? If I were an old-time philanthropist, I might not have needed to concern myself with whether the recipients of my 'charity' resented me for it. At least, it would never have occurred to me that they would.

Certainly a similar kind of 'ill-luck' in the problems which have to be faced confronts doctors when they attempt to act in the patient's best interest but find patients very much more vocal than they used to be. The problems which have to be faced are no longer just clinical (if they ever were): they are ethical as well, so that the very need to consider ethical questions raises issues of moral luck. This dilemma about paternalism versus patient autonomy, and what the moral luck paradox has to say about it, will recur in chapter 4 of this volume, on informed consent. In other ways, too, modern doctors are unlucky in the range of dilemmas which have to be faced: the rise of new technologies famously calls up new medical dilemmas all the time. The chapters of this book on new reproductive technologies, research and genetics all illustrate that point.

A very difficult set of issues concern *luck in character*, similar to Williams's category of *constitutive luck*: 'the kind of person you are, where this is not a question of what you deliberately do, but of your inclinations, capacities and temperament.'[16] Kant assumes that the good will may shine like a jewel in the blackest of circumstances, but what if having the good will is itself partially determined by luck? This dilemma radically undermines the notion of moral agency itself;

yet in some areas of psychiatric ethics – considered in chapter 8 – it is strikingly relevant. Similarly, to the extent that character and person-ality have a genetic basis, the problem of luck in character occurs there, as chapter 9 will explore. More broadly: the role of medical education, and of the Hippocratic oath, has been argued to be as much about inculcating the 'right' kind of character traits as about teaching knowledge or skills. What the 'right' kind of trait is has been seen to vary over time, from the 'reassuring' manner of the 'man in charge' to the modern-day emphasis on communication skills and consultation. But suppose none of this does any good at all? Suppose good or bad character is simply determined by luck?

Joel Feinberg argues that the Kantian attempt to drive responsibility inward, to intentions, the will or character, is ill-founded: we cannot evade the operations of luck so easily. As Margaret UrbanWalker puts it:

> Feinberg noted that it won't work to drive responsibility 'inside' to 'acts of the will', 'intentions', or 'character' as a way to evade the 'luck' of having other factors contribute to what you have done. For chance events, other people and circumstances can influence, even determine or avert, the occurrence of 'inner' states as well.[17]

The counsel of despair here would be that luck in character so radically undermines attempts to praise or blame that we cannot really have such a thing as ethics at all. The counter-argument put by Claudia Card is worth considering, however: character is shaped by how and for what we are held responsible.[18] We need not simply consign character to the unexplained and inexplicable realm of 'luck', to which ethical judgements cannot apply. Rather, ethical judgements also shape the development of character, in a reciprocal process.

Outcome luck: further considerations

The original sense in which moral luck was used was in relation to outcome luck, particularly by Bernard Williams. A recurring theme in this book is that the extent of outcome luck has been underestimated by philosophers, and that, although it occurs constantly in clinical practice, medical ethicists (and the clinicians whom they hope to assist) do not always recognize the paradox. When they do, in my experience of clinical ethics committees, they find the paradox helpful rather than irritating.

Ethicists have often failed to consider all possible outcomes, or have even assumed that the desired outcome is inevitable. Take, for example, the old saw about whether it is ethically justifiable to kill one person in order to save one hundred. The presumption is always that the hundred people will indeed by saved by the death of the one; but suppose they aren't? Even Williams himself can be accused of underestimating the number of possible outcomes in his well-known hypothetical case of Pedro and Jim.[19]

In this example, a traveller, Jim, happens into a South American market square where a captain, Pedro, is about to execute twenty Indians. Pedro offers Jim a chance to save all the Indians but one, whom Jim must kill by his own hand. If Jim refuses, Pedro says that all the executions will proceed; if he assents, Pedro promises that the other nineteen Indians will go free. Williams concludes rather grudgingly that the utilitarian answer – Jim should kill the Indian – is right in this case, although not for the conventional utilitarian reasons. As he puts it: 'The utilitarian is probably right in this case [but] that is not found out just by asking the utilitarian's questions.'[20]

Why Williams comes down in favour of Jim's killing the Indian is not the concern of my argument; I merely wish to point out that he has not fully considered what happens if things go wrong. It is all too easy – the stuff of B-grade films – to imagine Jim turning trembling to Pedro, smoking revolver in hand, and the camera panning onto Pedro's delighted grin as he takes the gun and shoots the first of the nineteen other Indians, whom he meant to kill all along.

Does this 'unlucky' outcome make Jim's decision wrong? A preliminary question that must be resolved is whether to call this outcome a mere matter of luck. First, 'unlucky' is too bland a term to describe the disaster that ensues. The more problematic matter, however, is whether luck means 'unforeseen contingency'. If so, then Jim, and Williams, cannot be castigated for failing to take it into account, for underestimating the number of positive outcomes. Here we can gain some purchase from Dworkin's distinction between choice and chance, or between option luck and brute luck. It seems inappropriate to claim that if all the Indians die, although Jim has decided to kill one of them in an attempt to save the others, it is merely a matter of brute luck or the operations of nature. Jim had a choice: this is a question of option luck. In reviewing all the options before making the choice, Jim, and Williams, failed to foresee a crucial possibility. In other words, I (and Dworkin) do not define luck as unforeseen contingency, merely as contingency.

A Kantian would assert that Jim's decision was wrong all along, regardless of the 'unlucky' consequences. More importantly, a Kantian *could* assert that the choice's rightness or wrongness is independent of the outcome. An ethical consequentialist, such as a utilitarian, would by definition be unable to do so.

Now possibly some utilitarians would argue that no additional diminution of welfare results from Jim's decision: all twenty Indians would have died in any case. But having failed to consider all the consequences should be a cause of self-mortification for any utilitarian strategy that incorporates probability assessments. This would include expected-value strategy, a common decision-theoretical model which advises the agent to choose among courses of action by multiplying the probability that an action will produce a desired outcome times the utility of that action, and its associated models, such as utilitarian economics, rational-choice theory in political science, cost-benefit analysis and quality-adjusted life years in health care economics. If the total number of possible consequences is not identified correctly, none of the probability estimates attached to any particular outcome can be valid. And this particular ill outcome should give pause to any utilitarian analysis that sets a negative value on giving additional pleasure to someone like Pedro. In that sense, Jim does make something worse happen by shooting the Indian. Certainly this unaccounted-for outcome should trouble Williams, since he sets a non-utilitarian, independent value on Jim's integrity, which has now been shattered for nothing.

In fact there are four possible outcomes in the Jim and Pedro example, not two:

1 Jim refuses to shoot the single Indian, and Pedro executes all twenty.
2 Jim refuses to shoot the single Indian, but Pedro, impressed by Jim's steadfastness and embarrassed by his own bloodthirstiness, repents and spares the others.
3 Jim shoots the single Indian, and Pedro liberates the nineteen others.
4 Jim shoots the single Indian, but Pedro breaks his promise. All twenty Indians die, as in scenario 1.

There are of course other possible outcomes, such as the cavalry rolling up in the nick of time, but these really are extraneous to the central agents, Jim and Pedro. Here I follow Williams's reminder to consider Pedro as an agent as well: 'While the deaths, and the killing, may be the outcome of Jim's refusal, it is misleading . . . to leave Pedro out of the picture in his essential role of one who has intentions and projects, projects for realizing which Jim's refusal would leave an opportunity.'[21] It may be questioned, however, whether Williams obeys his own injunction. By assuming that Pedro is incapable of options 2 and 4 or, more properly, by not considering Pedro sufficiently as an agent to see that options 2 and 4 are possible, Williams does in fact leave Pedro out of the equation, the terms of which he simplifies excessively. If Pedro is seen as an agent, whose mind Jim cannot fully know, then the problem of moral luck becomes all the more complex, insofar as the outcomes for which we may be responsible hinge not only on our own actions, or the actions of an impersonal nature, but also on the actions of other agents.

In later work Williams has dismissed the possibility of outcomes 2 and 4, regarding 1 and 3 as certain beyond reasonable doubt. But outcome 2 has occurred in several sieges involving the taking of hostages, when terrorists release their prisoners even though the authorities refuse to concede. It seems that Williams's impatience is directed at a more general political argument which suggests that 'the efficacy of the detestable action is more doubtful than the example supposes.'[22]

> This is a line often taken by those defending an absolutist position in cases of detestable actions extorted by threats made by hijackers and so forth, to the effect that the very character of the threat shows that one has reason to doubt the efficacy of giving in to it. Why should one expect such threateners to keep their promises anyway? As a *general* line of argument, this seems, bluntly, a cop-out.[23]

To me it seems that the 'cop-out' lies in attempting to write off possible outcomes which the moral agent ought to consider, assuming that she is considering consequences at all. However, at this stage of the book I do not want to commit myself to a general absolutist line such as Williams castigates. It may be that our disagreement is only over whether the Jim and Pedro example is one of those 'cases in which it is a reasonable bet that nothing is to be gained by giving in to threats.'[24] Even more narrowly, at this stage I merely want to suggest that it ought to be permissible to consider whether the Jim and Pedro example is such a case.

Suppose that outcome 2 does occur: Jim refuses to compromise his principles, and Pedro relents. The common response would be to admire Jim and to rejoice in the happy outcome. This casts doubt on whether Jim should abandon his integrity, but is the common response correct?

Intuition allows the actual outcome to make a difference to how we assess the agent's choice, but intuition also holds that moral choice is somehow impervious to how things turn out. We commonly do admire steadfastness, but would we call Jim mule-headed or callous if Pedro did not back down? This possibility may perhaps lie behind Williams's impatience with those who counsel against giving in to threats. Yet how can the character of the agent depend on the outcome? Character is meant to be more lasting than the rush and tumble of outcomes; we generally want to think that we are more than the sum of all the outcomes that occur in our lives. Thus the common response, that Jim should be admired for steadfastness if Pedro backs down, is incoherent. It exemplifies the paradox of moral luck, and we have already seen that the paradox of moral luck threatens the very notion of responsible agency. Yet the virtue of steadfastness, which would commonly be admired if Jim remained firm, also implies that there is a wholeness to the agent that cannot be diminished by ill-luck in outcomes.

Moral luck: how serious and genuine is the paradox?

The impetus in the debate between Williams and Nagel over moral luck is this inconsistency in common sense, and the broader, deeply disturbing question of whether outcome luck can threaten the concept of responsible moral agency. Both begin from Kant, as the source of the view that there can be a quintessential form of value, moral value, which is 'unconditioned'[25] – that is, free from external contingency. Both are also concerned to distinguish outcome luck from luck in character, antecedent circumstances, or problems which have to be faced. Their motive is to limit the potentially illimitable, although in this book I will be extending the operations of risk and luck beyond luck in outcomes. This is itself a risky strategy, although less so in a book-length volume. Listing all these ways in which moral agency appears to be subject to chance leads to a heightened sense of the possible threats to the very notion of moral agency from risk and luck.

> If one cannot be responsible for the consequences of one's acts due to factors beyond one's control, or for antecedents of one's acts that are

properties of temperament not subject to one's will, or for the circumstances that pose one's moral choices, then how can one be responsible even for the stripped-down acts of the will itself, if they are the product of antecedent circumstances outside of the will's control?[26]

We have already moved a long way from Kant's assertion that the good will has full worth in itself, even if it is totally powerless to achieve the good end. What is deeply troubling about the problem of moral luck is that it undermines the notion of the moral will itself, making it impossible for us to operate as ethical agents. Even confined to outcome luck, the paradox of moral luck is deeply troubling. As Nagel puts it:

> The inclusion of consequences in the conception of what we have done is an acknowledgement that we are parts of the world, but the paradoxical character of moral luck which emerges from this acknowledgement shows that we are unable to operate with such a view, for it leaves us with no one to be.[27]

If this is a genuine paradox, Williams agrees, then things really are quite serious, and there are only two possible resolutions, both unpalatable.

> One's history as an agent is a web in which anything that is the product of the will is surrounded and held up and partly formed by things that are not, in such a way that reflection can only go in one of two directions: either in the direction of saying that responsible agency is a fairly superficial concept, which has a limited use in harmonizing what happens, or else that it is not a superficial concept, but that it cannot ultimately be purified.[28]

Put another way, what is serious for medical ethics about moral luck is that it radically undermines the foundational, Kantian notion of autonomy.[29] Critiques of extreme advocates of personal autonomy have charged the autonomy view with a failure to count relationships in, to include 'the world' (in Nagel's terms) or 'the web' (in Williams's words).[30] But the opposite extreme apparently leaves no room for moral agency or personal autonomy at all; indeed, it seems to make the entire debate a nonsense, since there can be no such thing as ethics, medical ethics included, without a notion of responsibility and moral agency. If we are ultimately responsible for everything that happens in the world, then we are responsible for nothing.

But are matters really this serious? Is moral luck a genuine contradiction in terms, a true paradox, or has Williams overstated the problem? As a preliminary way of examining Nagel's answer to Williams, let us recast Williams's formulation of the moral luck dilemma in other terms, borrowing from Michael Zimmerman's method of restating the puzzle.[31]

1   A person P is morally responsible for an event e's occurrence only if e's occurring was not a matter of luck.
2   No event is such that its occurrence is not a matter of luck.
3   Therefore, no event is such that P is morally responsible for its occurrence.

Nagel, according to Zimmerman, denies the conclusion in (3) but accepts both premises (1) and (2), believing the paradox to be genuine (as indeed he must, to accept the first two premises but deny the resultant conclusion). Williams tends to accept the second premise while denying the first. If this is so, then Williams is not obliged to accept the paradox as genuine – still less to call for a complete overthrow of the Kantian ethical tradition, as he does, because he believes it is radically undermined by the paradox. In fact Williams goes so far as to doubt whether any doctrine of ethics, Kantian or non-Kantian, can resolve the paradox, although he holds out hope for Aristotelianism.[32] I suspect that Williams does accept the first premise as well. Certainly he is no less sceptical than Nagel, as Zimmerman's assessment would imply. In fact Williams presents himself as being more sceptical than Nagel about the possibility of an unconditioned form of moral value, untainted by luck.[33]

Both Nagel and Williams, however, appear to accept premise (2), which I think is actually the weakest link. *Although all events are a matter of luck, they are not all a matter of moral luck, nor are they all moral events.* Much of this book will be dedicated to examining this 'escape route' in relation to practical problems in medical ethics.

Zimmerman also proposes that we narrow the terms down; he believes that recasting the terms dispels the moral luck problem. Thus, if premise (1) is reformulated as 'P is morally responsible only if she or he was in restricted control of e', premise (2) cannot be upheld – if it is in turn recast as 'No event is such that anyone is ever in restricted control of it.' To reverse the procedure, premise (1) becomes palpably false if refashioned as 'P is morally responsible only if she or he was in unrestricted control of e,' while (2) is true if revised to read 'No event is such that anyone is ever in unrestricted control of it.' Thus the distinction comes to hinge on restriction over control.

In medical ethics, this recasting has a certain appeal. It builds in the rather unique way in which doctors' control is restricted not only by brute luck – the nature of illness – or by option luck – their own choices – but also by the choices of others – members of the clinical team, health care managers, patients and families. (In Dworkin's typology, brute luck probably includes the choices of others, but this manoeuvre does not really do justice to the decisions of others as moral agents.) Restriction over control is the everyday stuff of medical decisions. Yet it is palpably false, at least in law, to say that 'Doctor D is not responsible for failing to obtain informed consent, and for the ensuing battery to patient P, because she was not in unrestricted control over the course of events.' Much tension in medical ethics and law arises from the interplay of restriction and control, for example, in medical negligence, resource allocation, and research ethics. But even if the paradox is not so crippling as Williams believes, adding the refinement about restricted control does not dispel it altogether, I think.

To resolve the paradox of moral luck, we could absolve agents from responsibility for all matters beyond their ability to predict or control. But then we will wind up holding them responsible for very little. This is the strategy which Williams has pursued in subsequent work.[34] On a purely practical level, this tactic seems ill-advised in medical ethics: it leaves patients with very little protection and doctors with very little responsibility. On a considerably deeper level, it also denies the moral agency of doctors and makes them less complete people. On an intermediate level, it leaves doctors with no other guide than hindsight, which is of course no guide at all.[35] To understand why this is so, we need to examine Williams's examples, which illustrate his assertion that only success can justify an agent's decision under uncertainty.

Judgement from hindsight: Gauguin and Anna Karenina

Williams's first example is a fictionalized version of the painter Gauguin, who abnegates his responsibility to his wife and children when he abandons them to paint in the South Seas. Gauguin's failure as a painter would prove his decision to abandon his family was wrong in this rather opaque sense:

If he fails...then he did the wrong thing, not just in the sense in which that platitudinously follows, but in the sense that having done the wrong thing in those circumstances, he has no basis for the thought that he was justified in acting as he did. If he succeeds, he does have a basis for that thought.[36]

What can Williams mean here? Far from being so obvious as to be platitudinous, the rightness of Gauguin's action if he succeeds would seem quite hard to defend. If only success can justify a decision, but success is not certain at the time the agent makes a choice, there will turn out to be no basis but hindsight for judging whether an action was morally right or wrong. We do not generally think that agents are responsible for matter that they could only have known with hindsight. Therefore, if we take this view, we will not be able to hold agents responsible for very many of their choices.

Williams recognizes that Gauguin's success or failure cannot be predicted in advance; what he seems to be claiming is that only success can show us whether Gauguin had the sort of talent that could have served as a basis for the thought, at the time the decision had to be made, that his talent was the genuine article. In addition, he distinguishes between the factors intrinsic to Gauguin's success or failure and those extrinsic to it. Gauguin's decision is subject to luck on both counts, but only the intrinsic factors count in proving his decision to have been wrong.

> From the perspective of consequences, the goods or benefits for the sake of which Gauguin's choice was made either materialize in some degree, or do not materialize. But it matters considerably...in what way the project fails, if it fails. If Gauguin sustains some injury on the way to Tahiti which prevents his ever painting again, that certainly means that his decision (supposing it now to be irreversible) was for nothing, and indeed, there is nothing in the outcome to set against the other people's loss. But that train of events does not provoke the thought in question, that after all he was wrong and unjustified. He does not, and never will, know whether he was wrong. What would prove him wrong in his project would not just be that it failed, but that he failed.[37]

Williams is distinguishing between the failure of Gauguin's project and his failure as a moral agent. If things go wrong, they can go wrong in two ways, similar to the ways called option luck and brute luck by Dworkin. In Williams's view, Gauguin is not morally blameworthy if he abandons his family but fails to achieve his goal for reasons of brute luck. An event such as injury 'is too external . . . to unjustify him, something which only his failure as a painter can do.'[38] These external or extrinsic causes cannot always be predicted, but Gauguin could and should have sounded his ambitions and talents sufficiently to know whether he had it in him to be a great painter. If he failed because he did not have those qualities, then he could have been blamed. However, he may also have bad intrinsic luck, which is much more serious. The Gauguin who must assess his own talent as an artist, back in Paris, is one who has not yet sounded the full range of his artistic talents; he is in an important sense a different person from the Gauguin he might become if he goes to Tahiti. Since his knowledge is imperfect, and since he can know only in hindsight, as the Tahiti Gauguin, whether his decision as the Paris Gauguin was justified, the problem of moral luck in the decision he must make in Paris is serious and inescapable.

In chapter 6 I draw on a similar dichotomy in discussing how medical professionals should feel if they choose one patient over another for receipt of a scarce medical resource on the basis of the first patient's better prognosis, but if the patient who receives the kidney or the expensive procedure then dies. The doctors chose the 'wrong' patient, but it is inherent in the nature of prognoses that a certain proportion of them will turn out 'wrong', since they are statistical judgements. I present this example as a moral luck case in chapter 6, but I also suggest principles that would allow it to count as a project failure rather than a personal failure for the doctors as moral agents. Thus I do accept and draw on elements of Williams's analysis, but ultimately I agree with Nagel that it is too crippling.

Not all kinds of ill-luck are moral. Williams relies heavily on the idea that, if Gauguin does turn out to be a great artist, that outcome carries moral weight. But what if art has nothing to do with morality? In that case Gauguin's moral decision – and abandoning his family does incontrovertibly seem a moral choice – cannot be justified or unjustified on the basis of his artistic success or failure. Moral luck cannot enter into it: the decision is right or wrong from the start, regardless of outcomes, and no hindsight is required. Nagel's reply to Williams runs along similar lines:

> [Williams] points out that though success or failure cannot be predicted in advance, Gauguin's most basic retrospective feelings about the decision will be determined by the development of his talent. My disagree-

ment with Williams is that his account fails to explain why such retrospective attitudes can be called moral. If success does not permit Gauguin to justify himself to others, but still determines his most basic feelings, that only shows that his most basic feelings need not be moral. It does not show that morality is subject to luck.[39]

Gauguin's situation may be tragic if he cannot fulfil his genuine artistic talent without doing something morally wrong. But that is not the same as a genuine moral dilemma, in which both courses are morally wrong: for example, Sophie's choice, in William Styron's novel of that name, between allowing both her son and her daughter to die at the hands of the Nazis and choosing which one of them will live. Such moral dilemmas may also be subject to moral luck – Sophie cannot know in advance that the son, whom she has chosen, will die of natural causes in the concentration camps – or they may in fact be a subset of moral luck dilemmas.[40] But either way Gauguin's choice is not a moral decision, and therefore, by definition, it is not vitiated by moral luck. If he succeeds, he cannot justify himself to his abandoned wife and family by his success; if he fails, he is not more to blame because he has not succeeded – he was already to blame.

A similar criticism can be levelled at Williams's second example, that of Anna Karenina: it is not specifically about *moral* luck. Williams adds the (similarly schematized) example of Anna Karenina to that of Gauguin in order to illustrate the more typical case of someone for whom the locus of intrinsic luck is partly external. Here we begin to see important ways in which Williams's typology, intrinsic and extrinsic, differs from Dworkin's option and brute luck.

> The intrinsic luck in Gauguin's case concentrates itself on virtually the one question of whether he is a genuinely gifted painter who can succeed in doing genuinely valuable work. Not all the conditions of the project's coming off lie in him, obviously, since others' actions and refrainings provide many necessary conditions of its coming off – and that is an important locus of extrinsic luck. But the conditions of its coming off which are relevant to unjustification, the locus of intrinsic luck, largely lie in him – which is not to say, of course, that they depend on his will, though some may. This rough coincidence of two distinctions is a feature of this case. But in others, the locus of intrinsic luck ... may lie partly outside the agent, and that is an important, and indeed the more typical case.[41]

Williams takes Anna Karenina's suicide to be an admission that she has failed, not merely that her project has failed through some extrinsic factor – for example, if Vronsky had been killed in an accident. 'What she did, she now finds insupportable, because she could have been justified only by the life she hoped for, and those hopes were not just negated, but refuted, by what happened.'[42]

If we accept Williams's interpretation of the Anna Karenina story, grave paradoxes certainly ensue. Anna could not have known in advance that her affair would end badly, but she could only have been justified by its turning out well. What basis could she then have had for her decision about whether to leave her husband? This looks at first to be the problem about hindsight and responsibility that I identified before.

However, this example is really about what counts as an ethical choice and what agents are responsible *for*. The case of Anna Karenina cannot be the universal example that Williams thinks it is, because in Anna's society only women had to make such a choice. (Admittedly Anna is a schematized figure, as was Gauguin, but this excuse does not get round the problem of non-universalizability.) There is no moral luck in this example, because there is no genuine moral choice or responsibility.

Here the Kantian position would suggest that the genuine moral life must, by its nature, be equally open to all and its dictates be equally applicable to all. Because men were free of the strictures that required Anna to make a choice, because they operated under a much less restrictive system of responsibilities than did women in Anna's society, that system cannot be accounted a genuine moral system; nor can Anna's failure to live up to it count as a moral failure. Indeed, the fact that she had to make a decision at all is not evidence of a moral choice, but of victimization.

Anna had to decide between her lover and her husband and son. Her brother Oblonsky was allowed to keep both his mistresses and his home life. As the novel quite pointedly tells us at the very opening, 'although Oblonsky was entirely in the wrong as regards his wife, as he himself admitted, almost everyone in the house, even the nurse, [his wife's] best friend, was on his side.'[43] With a fine and deliberate irony, the novel begins with Anna persuading her sister-in-law to forgive Oblonsky for his latest dalliance. Williams seems to want to argue that Anna's affair was wrong from the start because it ended badly. Her brother's affairs don't end badly: are they any less wrong?

Williams does hone his analysis by noting that, once Anna left her husband, the relationship with Vronsky would have to bear too much weight. He calls her failure to foresee this an intrinsic matter. Certainly the novel's description of the lovers' scenes confirms that the relationship is overloaded, but that is only because society will not allow Anna to retain the marital relationship as well.[44] Although Williams calls this failure to forecast the extra burden on the relationship 'a truth not only about society but about her and Vronsky',[45] I cannot see that the occasion of the so-called moral decision would have arisen but for society's extrinsic laws and *mores*.[46] Still less do I agree with Judith Andre's contention that we would be right to praise Gauguin and blame Anna Karenina because 'the person who can correctly assess his or her chances of success is better formed than the person who cannot.'[47] This is to confuse acting ethically with being a clever technician. In any case, we do not know whether Gauguin judged the probability of success accurately or inaccurately: we only know that he succeeded.

Escaping from the paradox

The examples of both Anna Karenina and Gauguin can be construed as stories about something other than *moral* luck, and thus as no real threat. In most of this book I will be arguing along similar lines: that we can retain a notion of responsible agency, one which is not ultimately unsettled by moral luck, if we limit what agents are responsible *for*. Thus in chapter 4 on informed consent to treatment, I want to say that doctors are not responsible for the bad outcome of a procedure, provided they are not negligent, but that they are responsible for the prior duty of ensuring that the patient is informed of the likelihood of the procedure turning out wrong. In this way, and this way alone, responsibility for ill-luck in outcomes is transferred from the doctor to the patient. Although fully informed consent is something of a chimera, and a heavy duty in itself, obtaining as genuine and mutually communicative a consent as possible in the circumstances lessens the doctor's duties in the long run. Without such a notion, doctors would blame themselves for each procedure that turns out badly; no one can practise for long with such a mindset.

There is another possible escape route from the paradox which may strike a chord with many doctors, immersed as they are in history-taking: a narrative approach to the moral luck dilemma. This is what Margaret Urban Walker means, I think, when she writes:

> The agent is not a self-sufficient rational will fully expressed in each episode of choice, but is a history of choices...for whom episodes are meaningful in terms of rather larger stretches...We ought not to be surprised that...pivotal episodes which give sense to large segments are adequately judgeable only in retrospect.[48]

Chapter 9 will consider a developmental approach to responsibility, similar to Walker's approach. We will see there that such an approach is particularly relevant to medical genetics.

I have criticized Williams's two examples, but I firmly believe that medical ethics is full of genuine moral luck cases. It should be possible to stipulate in advance that good examples must involve agents who stake their moral success – not their worth as artists (or clinicians), their happiness in affairs foredoomed by social discrimination, or any other value – in advance on outcome luck.

Here is another such example: a research ethics committee that approves random clinical trials of a new drug on bowel cancer patients without informed consent. A patient with a prognosis of several years of active life dies two weeks later, because her bone marrow becomes irreversibly depressed in function after administration of the drug.[49] Let us suppose that no medical negligence is involved, that the drug was administered correctly but turned out to have side effects that no one could foresee. Is the outcome of the experiment the committee's fault? Or are there ways in which research ethics committees can limit what they are ultimately responsible for, and so avoid the paradox of moral luck?

It is important for doctors not to allow luck, risk and uncertainty in ethical decision-making to weigh so heavily on their minds that they are ultimately unable to act at all.[50] This is itself a risk, one that Williams rather too willingly embraces. Perhaps because I am not convinced about Williams's two examples, I am not persuaded by his fear of the 'final destruction' that occurs when Kantian strictness about the purity of the will is united with a utilitarian doctrine of negative responsibility. 'There is, at the end of that, no life of one's own, except perhaps for some small area, hygienically allotted, of meaningless privacy. Because that is a genuine pathology of the moral life, the limitation of the moral is itself something morally important.'[51]

Here I do agree with Williams, but I believe that he is now pointing towards a different path out of the maze. That is, rather than saying that we can have no meaningful conception of moral agency, he is claiming that we can have such a notion if we limit what agents are responsible for. This is close to my own hypothesis. An extensive catalogue of kinds of *luck* – such as the four suggested earlier in this chapter – is less crippling to the notion of moral agency than is a very broad notion of what counts as *moral*. No matter how deeply Gauguin feels about his failure as an artist, if he should fail, the intensity of that feeling does not itself make the failure a matter of ethics. If it is an ethical decision, that is because Gauguin breached his responsibilities to his family. They may or may not forgive him; they may cease to blame him, whether or not he succeeds as an artist. But if he stops being blameworthy, it is not because he succeeded as an artist; his original decision to abandon them remains a breach of responsibility.

Is this merely juggling with terms? I think not, in the example of Gauguin; but I also think that there will be cases in which the paradox of moral luck is genuine and troubling. Negligence is just such an area. Nagel gives the example of a lorry driver whose careless driving kills a child who darts into the road at the wrong moment. If the child had not run into the road, she would not have been killed; but, equally, the driver's negligence deserves blame. The question is how much blame. Here the law is somewhat equivocal, as is intuition. Many of us would blame the driver more if the child is killed than if she is not; yet this is to allow the operations of outcome luck to determine our moral judgements. If the driver is negligent, he is negligent not in the consequences but in his failure to drive properly, for which he can be blamed regardless of whether or not a child dies.

Perhaps we, and the law, do increasingly take this line in relation to drink-driving, but it does seem somewhat unrealistic to demand that anyone who exceeds the safe drinking limit should feel as deeply and profoundly to blame if he does not kill someone as if he does. Similarly, is the overworked junior doctor who prescribes the wrong dosage after an eighty-hour work week equally to blame if an experienced nurse pulls him up for his error, or if no one intervenes and a patient dies? It is unlikely that he would be disciplined by the General Medical Council in the first case, but should he be? If he and all his ilk were, would we eventually have no doctors at all?

On the other hand, it is surely correct to say that the drink-driver's negligence lies in driving while drunk, whether or not he causes an accident. He is being negligent in subjecting others' lives to unnecessary risk,[52] but what do we mean by 'unnecessary'? Exactly this question arises in many areas of medical ethics, particularly in research and psychiatry, and I will deal with it at greater length in chapter 8, as well as in chapter 4, which examines rationality and risk assessment in the context of consent to treatment. Virtually all our actions subject someone to risk, just as everything can be seen to hinge on luck, but in both cases these formulations are simultaneously insightful and too broad. To assert that we should never subject anyone to any added risk seems implausible, particularly in medical research; yet to use that as an excuse for piling on additional risks also seems an untrustworthy argument.

A firm critic of the notion of moral luck would have to assert that we should treat both sorts of case equally. How then can we explain the difference we draw between them? – except to say that we are wrong to do so. Norvin Richards, for example, claims that the ill-luck of the lorry driver who does kill the child essentially lies in getting caught. The driver who kills the child makes it clear to the world that he is a negligent driver; he should actually count himself lucky that he was not disciplined beforehand. Thus, luck does not affect one's responsibilities or deserts, only our knowledge of them.[53] Whereas Nagel accepts that moral luck is a genuine paradox (even if it does not apply to the wide range of events Williams wishes it to) and that the negligent driver who kills is more to blame than the one who does not, Richards asserts that the paradox is not genuine but merely a matter of confused thinking. Luck is more a matter of our epistemic position, our uncertainty and ignorance, than of what actually determines an agent's deserts. We must allow an irresponsible agent's luck in getting caught or not to determine to some extent how we treat him, since we are not omniscient. But that does not mean that ethics is radically undermined by luck in the way that Williams and Nagel claim it is.

This particular escape from the conundrum strikes me as rather cynical, although somewhat attractive, in that it logically calls on the practitioner to take seriously those examples of bad practice which are not detected, if only from self-interest. More deeply, it may be attractive insofar as it affords us a way out of the conclusion reached by both Nagel and Williams: that moral luck is a genuine paradox, imposing varying degrees of handicap on our ordinary assumptions about morality. A third possibility should also be considered: that moral luck is real – not merely a matter of fuzzy concepts – but that it is not a paradox. Rather, incorporating moral luck into our everyday assessments is not only possible but desirable. This is the virtue-centred view taken by Margaret Urban Walker,[54] which, together with similar proposals by Martha Nussbaum and Alasdair MacIntyre, will be examined at greater length in chapter 2.

2

The Fragility of Virtue and the Robust Health of Kantianism

Moral luck and virtue

If moral luck cannot simply be dispelled as a fallacy, and if it is a genuine paradox, the response may be to despair of the possibility of any solidly grounded, robust ethical system. This is indeed the course taken by Bernard Williams in his later writings. Since ascriptions of responsibility cannot evade the operations of luck, praise and blame become meaningless. (One may distinguish between holding someone responsible for a bad outcome and blaming her for it, in both a legal and a moral sense. If an autistic person or a person with learning disability commits an action resulting in a dire outcome, we may say that she was responsible in a causative sense, but we may choose not to blame her if her autism or learning disability was so extensive as to deprive her of a moral sensibility. However, in general I shall use the terms responsibility and praise/blame interchangeably.)

We commonly hold that people should not be praised or blamed for matters beyond their control; yet the typology of luck is so extensive that everything appears to be beyond our control. The most we can hope for, then, at least in Williams's view, is a system of ethics which is no more than consensual and no more than societal.[1] Any particular community may choose to honour certain ways of behaving and to blame others; indeed, it will need to do so in order to avoid anarchy. But we should not pretend that these purely relative, society-specific sets of values are anything like Kant's moral universals. The possibility of moral absolutes that transcend cultures or societies is thus obliterated by this interpretation of the moral luck paradox. In chapter 10 I shall return to the question of global ethics, and there I shall forcefully deny that the situation for global ethics is as dire as William's claims it to be. In chapter 2 I want to do something rather different.

We can see this non-absolutist train of thought manifested quite clearly in what has become known as 'virtue ethics'. While Kant would not himself phrase his dictum in terms of virtues, we might say that a certain virtue may indeed shine like a jewel in one society but be regarded as no more than paste in another. Although the classical predecessors of modern virtue ethics, particularly Aristotle, held that it was human flourishing and its requirements that dictated the virtues, modern virtue ethicists who claim that there is indeed such a thing as universal 'human flourishing' are often criticized for ethnocentrism or over-reliance on the rhetorical term 'human'.[2] Other virtue ethicists instead seek to ground the virtues for a society in what common sense for that society holds to be admirable.[3] Thus the paradox of moral luck, if taken to be genuine, should lead us to a radical pluralism of values: there can be no overarching, common moral concepts such as universal rights.

A community may be a community of profession as easily as of nationality – indeed, perhaps more easily.[4] If there is indeed a *telos* or aim of medicine, that in itself creates a kind of community. It is notoriously difficult to state what this aim might be: certainly it cannot be doing good to the patient even against the patient's will. Perhaps it might be maximal benefit with minimal harm or, above all else, doing no harm (*primum non nocere*). Whatever the agreed *telos*, if doctors, or nurses, can agree on certain virtues appropriate to it and germane to their professions, perhaps they can avoid the operations of moral luck in this manner.

Indeed, it is the traditional view of medical ethics that it is vocation-specific, and that its dictates are clear, unarguable, and rightly enforced by professional bodies such as the General Medical Council.[5] What is required in doctors, it may be argued, are certain reliable character traits which will take precedence over the physician's moods or own interests, and which are conducive to a good doctor–patient relationship.[6] These traits or virtues, such as benevolence, will probably predate the agent's decision to join the profession, and may well account for it, although they can be further developed with the right sort of medical education. What count as the virtues of a doctor, however, may be subject to change over time, as the profession agrees, as the law changes,[7] or as public pressure dictates. For example, the virtue of candour in physicians may well take on increased importance in the wake of the Bristol and Alder Hey inquiries into the taking of children's organs after death, without their parents' consent. Similarly, the virtue of 'caring' has acquired a pre-eminent status in much nursing ethics.[8]

This sort of argument has a certain plausibility and attractiveness. Provided that the profession takes its prescribed responsibilities sincerely, and does not just cynically use them as a justification for its social prestige, the vocational model is preferable to at least one alternative. That is the response to the operations of luck and risk which simply shrugs them off altogether. In the Alder Hey scandal of 2000, Dick van Velzen, the pathologist who amassed a large store of organs, including the brain of an eleven-year-old boy, appeared inclined to do just that. His attitude, at least as reported widely in the press, seemed very much akin to the response delineated more generally by Margaret Urban Walker, when she describes the one reaction we generally find intolerable when a bad outcome occurs but where the agent lacks entire control. That is the response which says:

> It's really too bad about what happened and the damage that's been done, but my involvement was just a happenstance that it was my bad luck to suffer. I admit my negligence (dishonesty, cowardice, opportunism, etc.) and accept such blame as is due these common faults. But it would be totally unfair of you to judge, let alone blame me for unlucky results and situations I didn't totally control, and stupid or masochistic of me to let you.[9]

Similarly, Professor van Velzen told Dutch television interviewers:

> I warned [Alder Hey] management from 1993 that from the ethical point of view it was a time-bomb. Now they are trying to describe me as a kind of Dr Frankenstein, just to get themselves off the hook.[10]

This claim seemed disingenuous in light of the evidence in the Alder Hey report that van Velzen suppressed discussion of ethical questions by his staff and assiduously amassed a collection of 6900 children's body parts. The Alder Hey pathologist might possibly have had our sympathy if he had pointed to the muddled position of the law, the ambivalent nature of the word 'tissue' in the consent form, the ostensibly higher goal of medical research, or the difficulty of explaining in detail to newly bereaved parents what tissue he required. But as Walker says of such a response as the pathologist actually showed, 'Even where we as third parties are disposed to be compassionate, fair-minded, and humane, we would be taken aback, and perhaps indignant. If our indignation were met by the agent with a cool reminder that we were conceptually befuddled about assessment and control, our estrangement would, I suggest, be aggravated rather than relieved.'[11] Integrity in both professionals and lay people seems to depend on feeling somewhat responsible even in situations we don't entirely control – that is, on recognizing the operations of moral luck but accepting that we may still be responsible, in some meaningful way, even when we do not entirely control the outcome. Rather like the Christian notion of grace, such an attitude potentially enables its holder to accept responsibility for outcomes ultimately beyond her control, without being destroyed by guilt.

If this line of reasoning is pursued further, it then becomes a virtue of the morally responsible agent that she recognizes her responsibility even when she does not fully control the outcome. That is simply part of being in the world, a fact about our limited human agency. (Many forms of Buddhism would also share this realization: that the boundaries between the agent's being and that of other agents, or of the world more broadly, are permeable and uncertain, so that the question of what I am personally responsible for is wrongly conceived.) Regardless of the outcome of our actions, this is the sort of person it is right to be. 'The truth of moral luck is that the rational, responsive moral agent is expected to grasp that *responsibilities outrun control*, although not in one single or simple way.'[12] This insight shares with Kantianism the recognition that we cannot control outcomes perfectly, but departs from Kant in stressing that nothing, not even the pure will, shines unadulterated in an impure world of impure agents. At best, we can try to cultivate certain patterns of behaviour that will, with further luck, become habitual. A virtuous person will have developed such virtuous habits and a virtuous character, through habituation and training, and that is the ultimate locus of responsibility. The question thus shifts from what it is right to do to what sort of person it is good to be.[13]

By focusing too exclusively on what it is right to do, rather than on what sort of person it is good to be, we make ourselves more vulnerable to the operations of luck and risk. If outcomes are beyond our exclusive control, as they usually are, but we are to be judged exclusively by the goodness of outcomes, there is nothing remaining that we can say to be truly under our control. But although we may also have initial good or bad luck in character, we may still achieve a greater degree of control over the sort of persons we become, according to this line of argument, through cultivation of certain virtues. One of these virtues will be the ability to see situations clearly,[14] without deluding oneself that one has any greater control than humankind can rightly expect. Thus the recognition of the operations of luck and risk is transformed from a stumbling-block to the ethical life into a precondition of it. In order to engage in the moral life at all, we must accept risk and luck; once we do so, however, our actions can count for something. As Walker says, 'In this picture, we are players within the complex causal set-up, where the price of our decisive participation is exposure to risk.'[15] Integrity is the virtue that accepts luck and risk, but remains steadfast despite their depredations.

This seems circular and fallacious, however, although initially attractive. If integrity is a virtue, it cannot be so universally, since by definition the virtues are a matter of consensus or established *mores* in each particular society; yet, if integrity is a precondition of the moral life, it must be universal to all ethical systems. Some virtue ethicists claim that the core virtues are effectively immutable,[16] but, more typically, virtue theories are particularistic rather than universal. (One corollary is that they therefore tend to be *status quo*, even nostalgic, as I shall argue of Alasdair MacIntyre in chapter 10.) Commonalities are hard to find, particularly on a global scale. Even within Western culture, the range of virtues allowed to women, in particular, has ranged widely from the limited notion of *sophrosyne* or restraint in classical Greece, through the daunting 'Cult of the True Woman' in nineteenth-century America, to a somewhat less gendered set in modern times.[17] More generally, how do we define a virtue in advance? – except in relation to some other system of values that tells us which are the right virtues.[18] It seems that integrity is being defined in advance as one of those right virtues; but on what basis?

There is also a risk, particularly in Walker's argument, of elevating the paradox of moral luck to a strangely desirable position, as that which enables or requires individual agents to exercise the virtue of integrity. Walker remarks that the virtues of integrity, lucidity and grace in the face of 'impure agency' 'are possible and necessary only for agents whose natural situation involves vulnerability to luck'.[19] Since these virtues are good, moral luck must also be a good thing. This reaction goes to the opposite extreme from Williams, who feared that the paradox of moral luck was so pernicious and far-reaching as to cast us into despair.

Furthermore, while virtue ethics may possibly deflect some of the dangers for a comprehensive notion of responsibility that are posed by moral ill-luck in outcomes, its emphasis on character leaves it open to luck in that particular department. Virtue ethics puts character first and action second, defining an action as right if it is that which would be done by a virtuous person in similar circumstances.[20] This seems to imply that, if anything 'shines like a jewel' in adversity of circumstances, it is the virtuous character: but we saw in chapter 1 that, if moral luck is a serious problem, it is a serious problem for character as well. One way out of that dilemma would be that taken by Claudia Card, who remarks that character is determined by those actions for which we are held responsible; that route, however, leads us out of virtue ethics and back to ethical theories such as Kantianism and consequentialism, which both focus more on rightness of actions. The only other way out seems to be equally snare-ridden for virtue ethicists. If it is a matter of luck whether some people's characters manifest integrity while others' personalities do not, then, if integrity really is a predecessor of all other virtues, manifesting the virtues will also be radically undermined by luck.

The fragility of goodness

One of the most comprehensive virtue-based approaches to overcoming the problem of moral luck has been provided by Martha Nussbaum, in her 1986 book *The Fragility of Goodness*. Nussbaum's critique of the Kantian approach also provides a useful bridge to a deeper elucidation of that perspective later in this chapter. I shall argue in this section that Nussbaum's elaboration of Kant is flawed, paving the way for my overall argument in this chapter: that the virtue approach is not in fact a necessary alternative to the Kantian perspective on moral luck. However, I will also recognize the merits of some aspects of Nussbaum's work, in order to leave open the possibility that some role for a virtue ethics approach may arise in certain of the applied chapters.

'If there remained only the good will ... it would sparkle like a jewel in its own right, as something that had its full worth in itself.' To Kant, the good will is implicitly beautiful, but, to Nussbaum, the good cannot be 'beautifully human' if it is distanced from chance.[21] Its fragility is precisely what lends an admirable and touching quality to human endeavour. In contrast, Nussbaum asserts, the Kantian attempt to create a risk-free ethics impoverishes that branch of human endeavour called acting well. This is particularly serious if the moral life is the highest branch of human endeavour, taking precedence over the more fully human life, as Nussbaum alleges it does in Kant. Nevertheless, Nussbaum recognizes that there is no reason to aim at moral excellence if it is not fully one's own, within one's own control – if it is inherently vulnerable to chance. 'The question of the human good' thus becomes: 'How can it be reliably good and still be beautifully human?'[22]

'Human excellence grows like a vine tree, fed by the green dew, raised up, among wise men and just, to the liquid sky.' Taking her metaphor for virtue from this quotation from Pindar, Nussbaum implicitly rejects Kant's 'jewel' parallel:

> The poetic image . . . suggests that part of the peculiar beauty of *human* excellence just *is* its vulnerability. The tenderness of a plant is not the dazzling hardness of a gem. There seem to be two, and perhaps two incompatible, kinds of value here.[23]

Still, the possession of reason is also part of human excellence: part of this particular plant's genetic blueprint is to develop the cutting hardness of a diamond. Nussbaum accepts the paradox of moral luck to the extent that she acknowledges that reason allows us to exercise some measure of control, making us less vulnerable to luck and chance than is the rest of creation. Through rational persuasion we have some hold over the actions of others, and even over our own propensity for irrational behaviours that may maximize 'option' illluck; through the application of scientific rationality we might likewise develop some control over nature, lessening the impact of 'brute' luck, to draw again on Dworkin's typology.

Notwithstanding, reason does not give us full control. The fragility of goodness – in Nussbaum's fine phrase – is confronted openly in Aristotelian philosophy and in the Greek tragic poets, according to her analysis.[24] Kantianism, however, refuses to recognize that the goodness or badness of character and the rightness or wrongness of actions simply do hinge on luck, on matters beyond the agent's control. What Nussbaum means by luck is both external contingency – everything that occurs through the agency of someone or something other than the moral agent – and internal character. With such a wide view of what counts as beyond our control, including good character, how then can we avoid moral paralysis?

Nussbaum insists that we must confront the vulnerability to chance of both right actions and good character. Kant's wilful blindness to this truth, she claims, together with what she views as the dominance of Kantian thought throughout the modern period,[25] has persuaded us that somehow tragic conflicts can be mitigated, if not avoided altogether. We delude ourselves into thinking that we can still retain a sense of responsibility as moral agents even when we are faced with two equally evil alternatives.

By contrast, Nussbaum claims, the Greek tragic playwrights recognized moral luck as inescapable, particularly ill-luck in the choices that have to be confronted. At Aulis, in the play by Aeschylus, Agamemnon faced a tragic choice between allowing the plague to continue among the becalmed Greek ships and sacrificing his daughter Iphigenia to placate the arbitrary will of Zeus. For Agamemnon to have been morally lucky, in the Greek view, would have been to have escaped this quandary altogether. Once it was visited upon him, albeit through no fault of his own, it was impossible for him to retain his moral integrity. No Kantian notion of a good will or pure intentions could have saved him from this ill-luck. The seriousness of 'tragic choices' in medicine will be further considered in chapters 5 and 6, on end-of-life decisions and resources respectively. As Bernard Williams says, 'There is no need of irrational gods, to give rise to tragic situations.'[26]

Here is a partial answer to the question of how we can avoid moral paralysis if character is not impervious to ill-fortune. It is possible for good character to endure such vicissitudes, but what it cannot endure, according to Nussbaum, is having to do things that are 'otherwise repugnant to [agents'] ethical character and commitments, because of circumstances whose origin does not lie with them.'[27] Tragedy is at its most disturbing when it depicts good people doing wrong things. However, they can retain a measure of their goodness and human dignity by explicitly recognizing that they are doing wrong things. This would be the opposite attitude to the 'shrugging it off' reaction castigated by Walker, the response which I thought I detected in the Alder Hey pathologist. There is a plausible honesty to this view, and a useful reminder for the medical profession. It is much more than a recommendation of hypocrisy, although it would still probably not be enough to satisfy the law or a professional review body.

To return to the example of Agamemnon: Nussbaum says that what is most evil about Agamemnon's decision to sacrifice Iphigenia is not that he does murder her, but that he becomes more and more convinced, as the play proceeds, that he should be praised for killing her. Because the sacrifice brings favourable winds – a form of good luck in outcomes – he is able to ignore the ill-luck in situations encountered that forced him to cause suffering no matter which course he chose. 'Agamemnon seems to have assumed first, that if he decided right, the action chosen must be right; and second, that if an action is right, it is appropriate to want it, even to be enthusiastic about it. From "Which of these is without evils?" he has moved to "May all turn out well." '[28]

But of course all cannot turn out well. Agamemnon has killed his daughter. The chorus blames him not so much for her murder as for his callous attitude towards it, for his lack of remorse. Without remorse, Nussbaum maintains, we cannot be said to be either fully human or genuinely responsible as moral agents. In this sense an awareness that acting well is vulnerable to the operations of luck, but that it is nevertheless incumbent upon us to act well upholds rather than threatens the ethical enterprise. This, too, I find an attractive view.

> Aeschylus has shown us how thoroughly, in fact, the pain and remorse...are bound up with ethical seriousness in other areas of life: with a seriousness about value, a constancy in commitment, and a sympathetic responsiveness that we wish to maintain in others and in ourselves...Without...acknowledgement of the tragic power of circumstance over human goodness, we cannot, in fact, maintain other valued features of our goodness: its internal integrity, its ongoing fidelity to its own laws, its responsiveness of vision.[29]

Because of our Kantian presuppositions, however, we are prone to distance ourselves from the Greek approach, Nussbaum asserts – to deny that some dilemmas simply are irreparably tragic. Instead, we see the Greek world-view, that moral value is vulnerable to luck, as primitive and fatalistic. To Nussbaum this is nothing short of a catastrophe for ethics, akin to the mythical one with which Alasdair MacIntyre begins his *After Virtue*. There, moral 'science' suffers a catastrophe before the academic history of ethics begins, 'so that the moral and other evaluative presuppositions of academic history [have] derived from the forms of the disorder which it (the catastrophe) brought about.'[30] In terms of the topic of this book, that would mean that the very attempt to evade the ravages of luck in ethics shows that we live in a sort of ethical Dark Ages, despite our pretensions to enlightenment and modernity. The pernicious influence of Kantian thought is largely to blame for our decline into a sort of moral barbarism, in Nussbaum's view.

Moreover, Nussbaum claims, the Kantian makes a watertight distinction between ethical value and other sorts of value, as the

Greeks, she says, did not. Not only does the good will shine like a jewel in its own right, having its full worth in itself; to a Kantian, its worth is also greater than that of anything else in the human sphere. This presupposition would lead the Kantian to a second, related conclusion about why Greek ethical thought was primitive: it did not even bother to distinguish between the ethically virtuous life and the good life for a human being. Rather, it conflated the two with its notion of *eudaimonia* or human flourishing, of which the virtues are manifestations. Both sorts of Kantian critique dismiss the classical virtue-centred perspective, largely because it appears to wallow in tragedy and chance.

> When the truth of these Kantian beliefs, and the importance of the Kantian distinction between moral and non-moral value, are taken as the starting-point for inquiry into Greek views of these matters, the Greeks do not, then, fare well. There appears to be something peculiar about the way they agonize about contingency, lamenting an insoluble practical conflict and the regret it brings in its wake ... It is as if they were in difficulties because they had not discovered what Kant discovered, did not know what we Kantians all know.[31]

Is this an accurate critique? Here is where I begin to part company from Nussbaum. Nussbaum essentially charges Kant with ignoring the dilemma of moral luck, with turning away from the myriad ways in which chance affects how things turn out, and focusing only on the purity of the will. Recall that the paradox of moral luck arises from the tension between 1) the way in which responsibility depends on some things outside moral agents' control and 2) our unwillingness to blame (or indeed praise) people for bad (or good) outcomes that were not in their control. Nussbaum accuses Kant of ignoring the first pole in the dichotomy. Yet it is just as likely that the moral luck paradox actually derives from a Kantian outlook, and from asking Kantian questions. In the next section of this chapter I endeavour to explain why this is so, and why I think that Nussbaum's critique of Kant is fatally one-sided.

Kantianism and moral luck

Let us begin with Kant's remarks in his *Lectures on Ethics* that a deathbed repentance is not a genuine act of conscience, because it has no chance of being carried over into practice.[32] No matter how pure the will may appear, it cannot shine like a jewel in this circumstance, because it cannot have an effect on the world. Kant wants conscience to have an effect on the world; does he also want the world to have some impact on the integrity of conscience?

In this section I want to defend Kant against the charge of ignoring moral luck (particularly luck in outcomes, although also to some extent luck in antecedents and luck in the circumstances that have to be faced). I also want to ask whether a Kantian solution to the paradox is actually possible, and indeed perhaps the most promising. The quotation from Kant with which I began chapter 1 shows that he is aware of the dilemma; whether the solution he proposes is sound remains to be seen. Because Kant proposes a solution does not mean that he ignores the problem: rather the reverse, although there is a tendency in Nussbaum to castigate him for ignoring the problem, precisely because he proposes a solution. My argument will be directed at Nussbaum's primary charge against Kant, then, but I also want to make some preliminary remarks about her second accusation: that Kant impoverishes the good life by narrowing it to the moral life. That sort of insularity Nussbaum presents as itself a moral fault, 'a ruthless simplification of the world of value which effectively eliminates conflicting obligations...refusal of vision.'[33]

What are the possible relationships between the moral life and the good life? Thomas Nagel distinguishes five possible forms of correlation between moral and other sorts of value.[34] One might want to add a sixth possibility rooted in feminist theory: the dualistic opposition between the good and moral lives is typical of the bilateral, dividing approaches that have dominated mainstream philosophy. I shall not deal at length here with this objection from feminist philosophers who suspect all dualisms,[35] but rather assume *in arguendo* that the relationship between the good and moral lives is a recognizable enough topic to merit discussion. If so, these are the five possible relationships:

1   *The moral life is defined in terms of the good life.* This position is attributed to Aristotle by Nagel. The two sets of values are not seen as equivalent: rather, the content of the ethical is dictated by background conditions for the good life, particularly the good life as appropriate for a certain social station (and, I would add, for masculine or feminine gender[36]).
2   *The good life is defined in terms of the moral life.* Both these first two positions deny that there is a conflict between good and moral

lives. Nagel reads the *Republic* as an elaborate and 'heroic' justification of this denial, seeing Plato as demonstrating empirically what Kant can only postulate: 'that moral virtue forms an indispensable part of the good for each person.'[37] The next two positions, however, admit that there is a disparity between good and moral lives.

3   *The good life overrides the moral life*: the view taken by Nietzsche, Thrasymachus in the *Republic*, and Philippa Foot in her later work. (Other characters in Plato's dialogues also voice aspects of this view, notably Gorgias, Polus and Callicles in the *Gorgias*.)

4   *The moral life overrides the good life*. Although Nussbaum identifies this argument as quintessentially Kantian, Nagel regards it as typical of utilitarianism and rights theories as well. The link between the two charges levelled by Nussbaum at Kantianism is highlighted by Nagel's observation that position 1 defines the good life as what is best for a particular individual, distinguished from others, we might say, by gender, age, social standing and other characteristics applied to individuals. Position 4 makes no such distinctions: it is concerned with the totality of humankind. As Nagel observes, 'Any coincidence between this [the good for all humanity] and what is best [for the individual] will be a matter of luck, or political and social arrangement.'[38] The importance of 'political and social arrangement' as an adjunct to luck is that it helps to explain cases such as Anna Karenina, which Williams misconstrued, as I argued in chapter 1, because he confused factors intrinsic to Anna's self-worth with those external social biases that doomed her project.

5   *Neither the good life nor the moral life consistently overrides the other.*

Let us consider position 4 to start with, since it is the focus of Nussbaum's secondary critique. It might actually be said that Kant is more aware than Aristotle of the operations of luck. The good life is dependent on the operations of luck, but the moral life, in Kant, is not, and, since the moral life overrides the good life, the importance of luck is minimized. Unlike the ancients (particularly Aristotle) Kant refused to accept a system of virtues in which the ability to attain praiseworthy behaviour depended crucially on station in society or other chance factors of birth. This is the relevance of his reference to the 'niggardly provision of a stepmotherly nature'.

Whether Kant did allow that participation in the ethical enterprise was limited by the chance factor of gender remains debatable: Susan Moller Okin, for example, asserts that, despite his impersonal terminology, Kant intends his conclusions to apply only to male persons.[39] On the other hand, Kant conceives of marriage as a contract between husband and wife, implying women's legal personhood,[40] although, equally, he is criticized by Hegel for assigning women, children and domestic servants a different and lesser formal legal status than men.[41] It may well be that, in relation to gender, Kant, like Locke, Marx and other 'malestream' philosophers, failed to follow his own logic thoroughly enough, but that the logic remains sound. (A somewhat less gender-biased application can be found in the more recent works by the self-described modern Kantian John Rawls, who has made some attempt to incorporate feminist critiques that he had not extended his logic sufficiently to include the accident of being born male or female.[42] What is also valuable is Rawls's insistence that intelligence is not a matter of desert or merit; therefore, under a system of justice as fairness, rewards should not flow from it.)

Nagel, too, comes round to the view that position 4 is probably sounder than the others, although he finds position 5 temporarily attractive. Clearly he disagrees with both Williams and Nussbaum, with their mutual preference for position 1. (Indeed, he might well accuse them of failing to distinguish 1 from 3.) What matters here is not so much his reason for approving the fourth view as his reminder that there are more than two possible relationships between the good and the moral lives. (Here, as in the Pedro and Jim example, ethicists have sometimes failed to consider all the possibilities.) If so, then the second of Nussbaum's charges against Kant is an oversimplification. Moreover, it is inaccurate, in Nagel's typology, to conflate Kant and Plato, as Nussbaum does. In the *Republic* Plato advocates philosophical thought because it is good in itself, not, as Nussbaum claims is true of Kant, because it is impervious to the vagaries of chance.[43]

What about Nussbaum's first charge against Kant – wilful negligence of the moral luck paradox? This is the more important accusation for the purposes of this section. It may be indicative that Nussbaum makes no attempt to differentiate between Kant's various ethical works, and in particular that she makes no reference in her bibliography to the *Lectures on Ethics*. The translator of the *Lectures*, Lewis White Beck, argues that it is in them, and also in the *Metaphysics of Morals*, that we glimpse the Kant whose lively conversation and striking way with words are said to have charmed audiences of students and enlivened drawing-room repartee. By contrast, Beck claims that, in the *Fundamental Principles of the Metaphysic of Morals* and the *Critique of Practical Reason*,

> everything anthropological and narrative or anecdotal, everything that would make perspicuous the relation of philosophical morals to the conduct of life, is there apparently sacrificed for an abstract intellectual articulation. It is no wonder, then, that Kantian ethics has since appeared to be forbidding in its intellectualism; to be rationalistic at the expense of emotion, habit, and institutions in the make-up of the good life; to have sacrificed all the graces for a few of the virtues... Only in the *Metaphysics of Morals* and the *Lectures* do we see what Kant never forgot, but what he expected his readers to remember even when he was talking of other things – viz., that the good life is more than mechanical obedience to the categorical imperative, that right action requires more than right thinking, and that man is more than a thinking machine.[44]

Failure to recognize this 'emotionally literate' side of Kant is commonplace. The usual presentation of Kant's system of ethics sees it as purely cognitive, narrow-minded, and lacking in human warmth. In somewhat more sophisticated versions, such as that presented by Laurence Blum,[45] Kant's concentration on the fortitude of the good will in adversity, as against the fragility of the emotions and virtues, leads him to ignore the greater reliability of the good emotions, despite their vulnerability to external contingency. In the long run, according to Blum, they are more reliable in producing right actions than is Kantian beneficence.

But how accurate is this 'dry-stick' view of Kant? To start, we must put paid to the notion that Kant's aim is to eliminate tragic choices. Nicholas White, in his critique of Nussbaum, emphasizes that we must separate Kant's view that there were no genuinely tragic choices from his position on moral luck.

> Although Kant seems to have believed that there are no genuine conflicts of duty, he was certainly not forced to that belief by his doctrine that the only genuine value is independent of contingencies. For he could have maintained that doctrine and still held that when a person is confronted with a genuine conflict of moral incommensurables, the goodness of his or her will is unaffected by making one choice or the other, so long as the decision is made in full consciousness of the existence of both obligations (which is not far from what Nussbaum herself seems to maintain).[46]

This seems a plausible line of argument. My own view is that Kant is not so much concerned with freedom from moral risk as with freedom of the will, and that the ultimately undetermined action of the will presents a sort of risk in itself – one that Kant does actually recognize. Nussbaum could in fact accept Kant if she had read him correctly. This position entails dismissing Nussbaum's criticism that Kant has simply ignored the way in which luck, particularly character and outcome luck, impacts on ethical choice.

Nussbaum seems to accept the commonly held view that Kantianism sets itself up as a risk-free system of ethics. Here she agrees with Nagel when he says, 'In Kant a course of action that would be condemned if it had a bad outcome cannot be vindicated if by luck it turns out well. There cannot be moral risk.'[47] To Nussbaum, a risk-free system of ethics is not worth having. Somehow the moral enterprise hardly seems worthwhile if it does not recognize how very deeply the rest of life is imbued with chance. This risk is so profound, she argues, as to threaten even the good will. Using the example of Euripides' *Hecuba*, she asserts that even good character may decay through chance reversals. This possibility is deeply repugnant to Kantianism, she says: in terms of 'a moral philosophy that speaks of the incorruptibility of the good will, sharply distinguishing the sphere of contingent happenings from the domain of the moral personality, itself purely safe against the "accidents of a stepmotherly nature" . . . this play tells dangerous lies.'[48] But the will is not the same as character in Kant: it is practical reason. A Kantian could perfectly well accept that good character is partly a matter of luck, just as intelligence is to Rawls. Both are normally considered achievements or personal virtues, but could equally well be partly matters of chance.

Actually, however, the Kantian moral enterprise is saturated with risk. One obvious way in which Kantian ethics deliberately opens itself to the full vagaries of chance is precisely that it refuses to excuse morally wrong decisions that happen to turn out well. (Nagel notes this, but does not present it for what it is, an assumption of extra risk.) Of course there are many cases in which bad judgement is rescued by good luck. I argued in the first chapter that Gauguin may well provide one such example: at the very least we cannot say that his judgement must have been good because the decision turned out well. Nussbaum actually agrees with this proposition when she says:

> We must avoid from the beginning a confusion between the assessment of the decision and the assessment of the deliberations that led to the

decision. It is perfectly possible for a person to have reached the better overall decision through a deliberative process that neglects certain valid claims; the decision will still, then, be correct – but not for the right reasons, and almost, as it were, by accident.[49]

However, Nussbaum regards the decision in the above case as still correct in some sense, even though correct by chance. The Kantian standard is stricter, and also more stringent than everyday attitudes towards blame and praise. No matter whether a wrong action turns out well, if we disobey the moral law 'we feel its power even when we are most defying it... The moral law itself, unlike any motive of desire, propels [us] onward to destruction.'[50] (Aristotle's view of tragedy was arguably quite akin to Kantianism in this regard: the tragic hero is propelled onwards to his own destruction by an inner dynamic, a tragic flaw that is punished by something like the moral law.)

The power of the moral law, in Kant, may thus appear at first to be utterly incompatible with the moral agent's freedom. None the less, the moral law, or the categorical imperative, obtains its legitimacy and force from agents' freedom. It alone is unconditioned by external factors. As Kant writes in the *Metaphysics of Morals*:

> The categorical (unconditioned) imperative views the action as objectively necessary and necessitates the agent to it immediately, by the mere thought of the action itself... and not mediately, by the thought of an *end* to be attained by the action... All other imperatives... are, one and all, conditioned... The *ground* of the possibility of categorical imperatives is this: that they are based simply on the *freedom* of the power of choice, not on any other characteristic of choice (by which it can be subjected to a purpose).[51]

It is precisely our freedom that enables the moral law to exist, in a two-way relationship. '[T]hough freedom is certainly the *ratio essendi* of the moral law [the reason the moral law can exist], the latter is the *ratio cognoscendi* of freedom [the reason we know that we are free].'[52]

Now there is obviously a link between my action being free and its being genuinely mine. 'Freedom is the power to will an end of action for myself... If my action is called unfree it is because there is a sense in which it is not truly *mine*.'[53] We have seen that Nussbaum – rightly, I think – denies that there is any reason for me to aim at moral excellence if it is not truly mine. So there will be a connection between my action being free and its being worthwhile. This is one reason why

I argue that Nussbaum is wrong to view the Kantian moral enterprise as unworthy of us.

There is another reason why it is simply incorrect to depict Kant as attempting to provide a risk-free ethics. In Kant the risk-free course, doing only what is required, carries no chance of blame, but also no possible gain in praise. 'If I do exactly what is required of me, the consequences are neither my fault, nor are they to my credit.'[54] It is the freedom of the moral agent that allows us to attribute responsibility. 'In a word, the key to the imputation of responsibility for consequences is freedom.'[55] Having said this, Kant then continues with the familiar dictum that the good will is not good because of its consequences; neither is it good because it is determined by externally defined duty. The good will can never claim to be simply following someone else's orders. Orders may be given either by an external authority, such as the law, or by an internal authority, namely practical reason. It is only the principles dictated by the latter that qualify as ethical pronouncements in Kant. An external law may have the same content as a genuinely ethical command, but we cannot claim to have behaved well if we obey the law out of frank compulsion.

Duty does not subordinate the will, although it determines the will temporally. Instead, duty is central in Kant because it is through the immediate perception of duty that the will realizes its unconditioned freedom. Paradoxically, Kant simultaneously presents duty as universal and also as entirely contingent upon each individual freely accepting it for himself. As Roger Scruton notes, 'Kant continued to regard the paradox of human freedom as unavoidable: we could never solve it through theoretical reason, while practical reasons assures us only that it *has* a solution.'[56] Freedom is also the distinguishing mark of an ethical choice as opposed to an action taken in obedience to the external law. As Kant elaborated the implications for responsibility and consequences in the *Lectures*:

> In the moral sphere compulsion has no place; no one can compel us to acts of kindness or charity. Thus moral omissions and their consequences can never be imputed, but legal omissions can. Conversely, moral acts of commission with their consequences can be imputed, but legal acts of commission cannot, since they are obligatory acts . . . I do not impute *in demeritum* the consequences of an action which a person is obliged to perform, because in such circumstances he has ceased to be free. He is responsible for the *factum* in itself but not for the *illegitimacy* of the *factum*.[57]

Here is another way of limiting what agents are responsible *for*, while preserving the meaningful notion of agency of which Williams despairs. Returning to the example of Agamemnon's tragedy, we could apply Kant's reasoning to argue that Agamemnon is responsible for killing his daughter, but not for the killing's being an evil deed. At first this conclusion looks puzzling: how can killing ever be anything but an evil deed? I do not wish to rehearse arguments about mercy killing or euthanasia here; let us assume *in arguendo* that killing is on the face of it an evil deed. The point is not so much whether killing could ever have any other moral content: it is rather that Agamemnon can be held responsible only for the bare action, not for the action's content. Zeus is responsible for that, presumably, if gods can be held responsible in the ordinary mortal way.

But precisely because Agamemnon is not to blame for the deed's illegitimacy, he should not try to justify what he has done. One might even go so far as to say that he is guilty only if he tries to justify killing his daughter as being somehow legitimate. This is of course exactly what he does do. There is a parallel here with the Alder Hey pathologist: his conduct is worsened by his trying to excuse it, by an apparently uncaring attitude. As Margaret Urban Walker claimed, this reaction is the one we find particularly insupportable in cases where a bad outcome has occurred due to factors not entirely within the agent's control. It is very common indeed for families to launch complaints and medical negligence actions not because of the bad outcome itself, but in order to force the hospital and consultant to take some responsibility for their actions, to apologize.

What does Kant's view offer as an alternative? In subsequent chapters I shall focus on the way in which a Kantian perspective allows us to limit what we are responsible for, so long as we take full responsibility for that limited responsibility. This will be the crux of the chapter on informed consent, for example. Kant also asserts that we can be held responsible for setting events rolling through actions that we could control, although not necessarily for all the consequences of those actions.

> Whatever appertains to freedom can be imputed to us, whether it arises directly through our freedom, or is derived indirectly from it. A drunken man cannot be held responsible for his drunken acts; he can, however, for his drunkenness. The causes which make it impossible to impute responsibility to a person for his actions may themselves be imputable to him in a lower degree.[58]

Not only is there a connection between my action being free and its being truly mine: there is also a link between my action being free and its being invulnerable to moral luck. What can be said to belong to the drunken man, and what he can be held responsible for, regardless of whether or not his drunkenness causes any actual harm to others, is his decision to drink heavily in the first place. Similarly, what a medical or nursing professional who breaks professional codes can be held responsible for is not necessarily a bad outcome resulting from the transgression: she may get off lucky, or there may be other contributory causes to the bad outcome. It is breaking the code itself. Indeed, one might argue that this is the exact purpose of professional codes: to limit the operations of moral luck. What the General Medical Council's disciplinary jurisdiction covers is not only the cases in which dire outcomes do occur but, more broadly, cases of disregard of professional responsibility to patients. Even more strictly, nurses in the United Kingdom may be disciplined for a wide variety of forms of 'professional misconduct' without even the requirement that the misconduct should be 'serious', as applies to doctors.[59]

The Kantian precept above is apposite to an example given by Nagel, that of a drunken driver who swerves dangerously onto the pavement. Now Nagel does not actually take a Kantian line here: he asserts rather that the driver is morally lucky if there are no pedestrians on the pavement, and morally unlucky if there are. As he notes, 'If there were, he would be to blame for their deaths, and would probably be prosecuted for manslaughter.' However, he may well be prosecuted for reckless or dangerous driving; the law recognizes a degree of responsibility here, even if a lesser degree. Arguably, it should not be a lesser degree. Intuitively we do think that the driver should say to himself, 'I could have killed someone', and stop combining alcohol and driving. We do blame him whether or not an accident occurs.

This Kantian way out of the paradox of moral luck, which common sense has created, is itself consistent with common sense. Kant would probably have regarded this consistency as a considerable virtue. In dismissing the criticism that the *Fundamental Principles of the Metaphysic of Morals* contained 'no new principle of morality in it, but only a new formula', Kant riposted: 'Who would want to introduce a new principle of morality and, as it were, be its inventor, as if the world had hitherto been ignorant of what duty is or had been thoroughly wrong about it?'[60]

In rejecting the usefulness of Kantian precepts such as the one above, and in taking the 'dry-stick' view of Kant as someone who tried to seal himself and his philosophy off from the world of chance and the emotional life, Nussbaum overemphasizes the negative conception of freedom, which does sometimes occur in Kant at the expense of the more positive concept. Roughly speaking, the negative reading is freedom from sense-impulse, which can affect free choice but which cannot determine it. The positive concept, which I view as more important, is the power of pure reason to be practical in and for itself, without dependency on some externally given law.[61] The centrality of this positive concept of freedom is illustrated in this quotation from *The Metaphysics of Morals*:

> In reason's practical use the concept of freedom proves its reality through practical principles which, as laws of a causality of pure reason which is independent of all empirical conditions (of sensibility as such), determine choice and prove the existence in us of a pure will in which moral concepts and laws have their source.[62]

Ironically, the 'dry-stick' view of Kant may also be influenced by what is actually most personal and revealing in Kant's writing: the struggle against odd inclinations and chance passions, on the grounds of their irregularity, their vulnerability to contingency, rather than their content. Even the virtues are vulnerable, suggesting an awareness of luck in good character – and creating an unlikely kinship with Nussbaum's analysis of *Hecuba*. Moral innocence, Kant notes wryly, would be 'glorious' but for the high probability of its downfall.

> Innocence is indeed a glorious thing; only, on the other hand, it is very sad that it cannot well maintain itself, and is easily seduced. On this account even wisdom – which otherwise consists more in conduct than in knowledge – yet has need for science, not in order to learn from it, but to secure for its precepts admission and *permanence*.[63]

Similarly, accepting favours is a breach of one's duty to oneself, because there is always a risk that the debt will be called in, in some unpalatable and unforeseeable way. This thrust towards controlling the unpredictable and unstable is a continual theme in Kant, as in this quotation from *Religion within the Limits of Reason Alone*:

> When incentives other than the law itself (such as ambition, self-love in general, yes, even a kindly instinct such as sympathy) are necessary to determine the will to conduct conformable with the law, it is merely

accidental that these causes coincide with the law, for they could equally well incite its violation.[64]

Yet Kant also warns us that hedging one's emotional bets cannot alone constitute the ethical life:

> Moderation in the affections and passions, self-control and calm deliberation, are not only good in many respects, but even seem to constitute part of the intrinsic worth of the person; but they are far from deserving to be called good without qualification, although they have been so unconditionally praised by the ancients.[65]

This self-restraint 'so unconditionally praised by the ancients' – ironically enough, for Nussbaum's argument – is too dry a virtue to be called 'good without qualification'. Despite Nussbaum's argument to the contrary, I believe that Kantian ethics can be 'beautifully human'. Kant, it seems to me, does take account of the full range of human needs and attitudes; he does not want us to close ourselves off through an obsessive frugality of the emotions and continual scrutiny of our motives. In particular, he is fully aware of our need for a motivating force to obey the Categorical Imperative, beyond that which can be provided by logic alone.

> Morality consists in this, that an action should arise from the impulsive ground of its own inner goodness . . . That it is so is well appreciated by the understanding. Nevertheless, this impulsive ground has no driving force . . . But we should be on our guard against becoming hypercritical about it, against probing too deeply into its incapacity to attain moral purity. Those who are forever on the look-out for moral impurities in their actions tend to lose confidence in their ability to do good and moral actions.[66]

This is a pragmatic, self-aware counsel with a great deal of applicability in medical ethics. Moral burnout is as much a risk for the conscientious doctor as is clinical burnout. What Kant warns us against here is the loss of confidence which results from too much introspection, and too stringent a sense of responsibility. One such temptation to the morally sensitive is awareness of the myriad ways in which luck can undermine our best intentions and threaten us with responsibility for outcomes we cannot control. What Kant offers us here is a counsel of caution and humanity, 'against probing too deeply into [our] incapacity to attain moral purity'.

Perhaps it is in fact a Kantian kind of virtue, a proper humility, not to become too obsessive about one's responsibilities? This would be a surprising conclusion, in light of the general opinion of Kant, but it would suggest some common elements between virtue ethics and Kantianism. I shall suggest in the next chapter that these similarities are even more pronounced in contrast to ethical consequentialism, particularly utilitarianism. There, I shall argue, obsessiveness knows no end and the problem of moral luck no bounds.

3

Utilitarianism and Luck
in Outcomes

Although I have denied that Kant strives to create a risk-free system of ethics, I do not deny that moral luck looks at first to be particularly paradoxical for a Kantian. A Kantian is concerned primarily about the state of her own will, but how can a will be durably good if its goodness is subject to factors beyond the agent's control? Against Nussbaum's assertion that Kant deliberately chooses to ignore the myriad ways in which moral agents are subject to chance and risk, in order to preserve the integrity of the good will, I have argued that Kant does in fact recognize something like the moral luck paradox, and that he offers at least a partial resolution of it. This solution can be achieved through limiting what agents are responsible for, while retaining a strict notion of agency.

Let us recapitulate at this point what those factors beyond the agent's control might be, in terms of the categories of moral luck introduced in chapter 1:

- luck in outcomes, subdivided further into 'brute' and 'option' luck
- luck in antecedent circumstances
- luck in the problems that have to be faced
- luck in character.

Whereas chapter 2 concerned mainly the latter three forms of moral luck, particularly luck in character insofar as it covered virtue ethics as well as Kantianism, this chapter will concern primarily utilitarianism's position on the question of luck in outcomes, concentrating on what Dworkin would term option luck. As a form of ethical consequentialism, utilitarianism, which measures the value of an action by the amount of welfare produced as its consequence, can readily be seen to be most relevant to outcome luck.

Now because utilitarians do emphasize consequences rather than conscience, it might be argued that the dilemma of moral luck does not exist for them. If this were true, it would be better than Kant's partial resolution of the problem: it would abolish the problem altogether, or at least deny that the paradox is genuine and germane to ethics. Arguably, it is only by asking Kantian sorts of questions about the integrity of the good will, not the value of consequences, that the problem of moral luck arises at all. Moral luck then looks like some sort of arcane Kantian obsession that can easily be eliminated by converting to utilitarianism. But are matters so simple?

Perhaps this might be a good time to restate the paradox, which depends on a dichotomy between the outside world and what is defined as the locus of moral worth in the individual agent. If right and wrong, as well as good and bad, pertain purely to consequences, rather than to the will, it looks at first as if the problem of moral luck cannot arise. The dichotomy should no longer exist, because the locus of moral value has shifted from the agent to the outside world. Since the paradox of moral luck results from this tension between individual responsibility and determination by things outside the agent, consequentialists might argue that they are able to eliminate the paradox.

Commonsense judgement holds people responsible for their actions partly according to how those actions turn out. Yet common sense also maintains that people are not responsible for matters beyond their control. Much of how things turn out is inevitably beyond agents' control. It is possible to resolve this, the paradox of moral luck, by ceasing to hold people responsible for what is beyond their control, but then we may not wind up holding them responsible for very much. This is essentially the line that Williams has pursued, increasingly abjuring any notions of ethical values as supreme values and of ethical systems as universally binding. The radical value pluralism that results will be examined at greater length in chapter 10.

What I want to concentrate on here is the issue of whether such a radical response is necessary: whether utilitarianism can offer an alternative way out of the paradox, or even dispel the paradox altogether. I conclude that it cannot: that moral luck is not a peculiarly Kantian fixation, even though the dilemma appears to arise by asking Kantian questions about the moral integrity of the agent. It seems at first that consequentialism does not have a problem with moral luck, although of course it does concern itself with how to make the optimal choice under conditions of risk and uncertainty. (These questions also bear on rationality in decision-making, and they will be aired to some extent in this chapter, although I shall not go through the vast and often technical literature on rational choice theory in economics, philosophy and political science.[1] Rationality in decision-making will be further dealt with in chapter 4, on informed consent to medical treatment.) However, I shall argue that moral luck is also a problem for utilitarianism, and for consequentialism more generally. The reason why this is true relates to how consequentialism has defined what kinds of outcomes the agent is responsible for, and this in turn relates to probability and risk.

Actual consequences

To ascribe responsibility on the basis of consequences inevitably raises the question of whether the agent is responsible for the *actual* or the *potential* consequences of her actions. If the answer is the actual consequences, we have not evaded the problem of moral luck at all. The rightness or wrongness of my decision will still depend on some matters beyond my control, if matters do not turn out as I had intended or foreseen. (I shall not distinguish between the two at this point in the argument.) If we still want to retain some conception of responsibility and agency, this creates a temptation to think in terms of potential consequences, which are normally translated into the likelihood of each outcome and its desirability, or probability and utility.

Whether it is actual or probable consequences that are most ethically relevant is a debate that goes back at least to Bertrand Russell and G. E. Moore, as discussed by C. D. Broad in 'The doctrine of consequences in ethics'.[2] Broad thinks that the Moore–Russell controversy suggests that even ascribing responsibility by actual consequences requires probabilities to be taken into account. Although Moore held, against Russell, that it was actual consequences that mattered, he was also compelled to introduce probability in the end, according to Broad. This is not the main point at the moment, however: rather the question is whether a form of consequentialism that thinks solely in terms of actual consequences – whether or not it has to incorporate probabilistic reasoning – is not just as vulnerable to the paradox of moral luck as Kantianism has been alleged to be.

It does appear that Russell was aware of how reliance on actual consequences as the touchstone somehow lessens the moral agent's control and may make it hard for us to know just what the agent could rightly be held responsible for. This is essentially the moral luck problem. Using probable rather than actual consequences as the guide has the advantage 'of making objective rightness independent of unforeseeable circumstances'.[3] Now, not controlling is broader than not foreseeing: foresight is at best a minimal sort of control. I shall need to distinguish between the two later on in this chapter, when I come to consider rationality at somewhat greater length. But there is a germ of a moral luck argument in Russell's realization here, and one that appears to work in favour of potential rather than actual consequences. (I shall return to consequentialisms of potential consequences in the second section of this chapter.)

In contrast, Moore is not too bothered by the dilemma of moral luck. Being judged by the actual consequences, he asserts, will not turn out to be intolerably harsh, because we ought to distinguish what it is right to do from what it is right to praise. It may still have been right for me to perform an action that resulted in an adverse outcome beyond my control, even though I am unlikely to win any praise for it. Furthermore, *rightness* refers only to consequences, according to Moore, but we may still say that the agent's choice was *good* even if the consequences turned out wrong. Although Broad calls Moore's formulation generally more plausible than Russell's, his preference for Moore's position does not extend to the claim about praise and blame. 'This supposition is not necessarily true: A's praise or blame of B's act is a second act, and like all others, its rightness or wrongness must be judged by its own consequences, and not by those of B's act.'[4]

So Broad is unwilling to allow Moore this evasive action, although perhaps because Broad himself does not fully recognize how deeply the moral luck problem would affect a consequentialism based on actual outcomes. He is blithely willing to accept that, 'since the rightness of your action is at the mercy of all that is going to happen in the universe throughout all future time, there is no reason to expect better results from conscientious acts than from the most stupid and biased ones.'[5] This conclusion is hopelessly demoralizing: to a consequentialist, the point of making conscientious decisions is precisely to obtain better results, not to make the decision dutifully or in accordance with prior principles. If there is no reason to expect better results from conscientious acts than from stupid ones, there can be no reason – at least not in consequentialism – to make ethical choices in a conscientious manner. (There would be reasons in Kantianism, of course.) It is therefore hard to see how Broad's formulation could motivate right action; he cannot ignore ill-luck in actual outcomes so easily.

Broad's main reservations about relying on potential outcomes concern Russell's alleged mingling of actual and probable consequences, with disastrously confused results. As Broad puts it,

> It is not clear whether the objective rightness of an act depends on the actual value of its probable consequences, or the probable value of its actual consequences, or the probable value of its probable consequences. All we are told is that it does not depend on the actual value of its actual consequences.[6]

Of course this does not defend the actual consequences position against the moral luck problem: it merely criticizes Russell's particular formulation of the potential consequences line. Is it impossible to formulate a consequentialism of actual outcomes without encountering moral luck dilemmas? I have suggested so far that the answer is probably yes, but A. N. Prior's work provides additional grounds for doubting that an actual consequences form of utilitarianism can work.[7] His argument bears on moral luck, although it is not couched in those terms – rather, in those of a different paradox.

Moore maintains that it is our duty to perform that action which actually produces the best total consequences, of all available alternatives. However, Prior calls it logically impossible to determine the contents of that duty – not only because we lack the necessary predictive powers, but also because Moore is making paradoxical assumptions about control. No such best package of outcomes can exist unless determinism is total, but of course if determinism is total and free will is non-existent, we cannot be said to make ethical choices at all. The total future of the world depends on how other agents choose, too – not just on how I choose.

There is a distinction between the uncertainty introduced by our inability to control many of the decisions made by others and that entailed by our lack of knowledge of the future. The first is certainly part of the paradox of moral luck, but the second also enters into it. Prior regards the first as the principal difficulty for a consequentialism of actual outcomes. The second, he says, 'is only part of the general problem of "duty and ignorance of fact", which has nothing specially to do with utilitarianism, and [which] was allowed for by Moore anyway.'[8] But surely our lack of knowledge of the future is a practical problem for a consequentialism of actual outcomes?

One other well-known consequentialist, at least, seems largely unbothered by it. Richard Brandt stakes a great deal on our being able to know the rational or best action at the time we make our decisions. Moral luck is not a quandary for him, because he believes that we can control the outcome of our choices at least minimally, through foresight. Nor is he disturbed by Russell's doubts about using actual consequences as the touchstone of right action, a scepticism based on the vulnerability of actual outcomes to external factors. Brandt appears quite happy to judge by actual rather than possible outcomes in many of his examples:

> It is a fact that people are uncomfortable if a decision they make turns out to have distressing consequences, when they know it would have been avoided by fuller or more careful reflection. For instance, if one buys a car which turns out to hold the road poorly and to consume large quantities of petrol, and if one knows one could have anticipated these facts by perusing an easily available copy of *Consumer Reports*, one is quite annoyed with oneself. Now a rational action is by definition one which avoids all mistakes deriving from inadequate reflection.[9]

This position seems hopelessly naïve, and excessively demanding. The very best-informed consumer can only find information in consumer magazines that bears on statistical aggregates, groups of all cars of that particular year and model, obtained by testing a statistically valid number of vehicles chosen at random from that class. Even assuming that these procedures can be followed to the letter, the report will only be correct in the long run. Nothing stops it being right in the long run if the particular car I have the misfortune to buy turns out to be the odd 'lemon'.

Brandt defined a rational action not as one that took the correct background data into account, but as one which *avoids all mistakes deriving from inadequate reflection*. Of course we could engage in sophistry by claiming that a decision that turns out wrong must automatically reflect inadequate reflection and that, conversely, a decision that turns out well automatically reflects proper forethought. Failing that stratagem, however, a consequentialism of actual outcomes like Brandt's is obsessively unforgiving of mistakes.

Recall that the dilemma of moral luck concerns the simultaneous common sense requirements that we should be held responsible only for actions that we can control, and that we should be held responsible for our actions partly according to how they turn out. If Prior is right, a consequentialism that attributes responsibility according to how things actually turn out radically extends what we are responsible for, despite our inability to predict events except, at best, statistically, and despite our usual inability to control fully the actions of other agents. A doctor who judges herself by whether things have actually turned out right will land squarely in the middle of the moral luck paradox, and will frequently have ample grounds for remorse. (I shall return to questions of remorse and responsibility in the third section of this chapter.)

Potential consequences

Can the paradox of moral luck be avoided by using potential or probable consequences as our guide for action? Prior prefers to leave agents responsible for a broad range of outcomes, but not for *actual* consequences. We may have to be content to consider as our duty that action which will *probably* engender the most desirable total consequences, he says. However, this position also leads to difficulties: for example, probabilities must be conceived as having an objective existence, Prior stipulates. It is not enough that we believe the consequences of an action are likely to a certain degree: they must actually be probable at that level of magnitude. After all, what affects other people is the outcome, not my estimate of it. But on this argument it would be actual consequences that count after all, since they are what affect other people.[10] In fact a consequentialism of probable consequences seems to be allowing its adherents a rather Kantian excuse, that they acted with good intentions or a good will. Believing that in the long run such-and-such an action will produce good results, based on a favourable balance of probabilities, counts as having a good intention. Yet normally consequentialists are quite scathing about the excuse of good intentions. For example, utilitarian medical ethicists frequently criticize the doctrine of double effect as applied to administering high doses of pain relief, with the primary intention of relieving pain but the foreseen (although not intended) effect of killing the patient.[11]

Although utilitarians typically present their approach as hard-headed and realistic,[12] there are real difficulties about what probabilities actually represent – in fact, whether they represent anything real at all. Utilitarianism relies upon the notion of expected value, that is, the calculus of probability times utility. Yet as Broad says about expected value, '[there is] no reason to think that the notion of mathematical expectation is really a measure of anything in this world.'[13] The real culprit is probability. Utility may be difficult to measure – as in the well-known difficulties in calculating QALYs, quality-adjusted life years, of assigning a mathematical value to the patient's assessment of a particular outcome's value, lying between 0 for death and 1 for perfect health. However, at least that value represents something definite, the patient's own assessment of her preferences for particular outcomes in her own situation. It is not so clear that a probability represents a concrete something; however, I do not wish to go into complicated issues of epistemology. Rather, I want to introduce some of the well-known paradoxes of probability, in order to demonstrate that the 'probable consequences' route out of the paradox of moral luck leads only into further paradoxes.

I said before that we need to distinguish uncertainty born of ignorance from that stemming inevitably from the freedom of other agents. A concentration on probable consequences looks at first as if it can lessen much of the first kind of uncertainty, through the statistical discipline of probability interpretation. (However, even if this is true, it does not answer Prior's objections about control of others' actions.) Of course, we do, incontestably, use probabilities in ordinary prudential decisions. So why should we deny ourselves their help in moral choices? Aside from the arguments within statistical theory about whether probabilities are objective or subjective – and as Broad argues in relation to whether mathematical expectation represents anything real, these are substantial philosophical matters, not just technical questions – there are grave questions about using probabilities as the touchstone for right action.

Two sorts of questions arise. The first has to do with mistakes in moral mathematics, the second with incommensurability of moral value. Both sorts of question are illustrated in the following example, but I shall need to separate them out in elucidating it. Broadly, however, the point of the example is that we cannot improve matters by trading in one paradox for another. I want to suggest that the paradoxes of probability are no less crippling than those which moral luck presents, and that some utilitarians have been insufficiently aware of their imperviousness to better methods of calculation.

Consider a typical probability, that of dying in a motor vehicle accident. Let us say that the risk is 0.0027, or 27 deaths for every

10,000 people per year.[14] These deaths constitute a statistical certainty, within the limits of the appropriate degree of confidence. Of every 10,000 people, 27 could 'certainly' have expected to die in road accidents that year, although of course no one knew which 27 would die. Yet the group total is certain, and indeed is derived by taking those who did die in road accidents as a proportion of the total population. Now let us consider a probability derived with similar certainty from actual figures, although in a hypothetical example.[15] The point here is that there is no quibble about whether the probability is accurate, and no improvement in the paradoxes illustrated by the example could be made by obtaining the initial probabilities in some more accurate fashion.

Twenty-five prisoners are exercising in a yard, under the surveillance of a lone guard. A solitary witness, who is too far away to identify any of the prisoners, sees the guard – recognizable by his uniform – trip and fall, knocking himself out. After huddling together for a moment, the prisoners separate. One hides in a shed in the corner, while the other twenty-four fall on the guard and kill him. Then the last man re-emerges and mixes with the other prisoners. The rest of the prison guards rush into the yard, where they find their dead colleague and the twenty-five prisoners. How many, if any, will be found guilty of murder?

None, says the originator of the example, Charles Nesson: no jury would convict any of the prisoners. To do so would be equivalent to announcing that the jurors believed a probability of 0.96 (24 out of 25) to constitute guilt beyond a reasonable doubt, which is the standard in criminal prosecutions. Such a conclusion would be detrimental because doubt serves a social purpose: the public can defer to jury verdicts only if they are not couched in such bald and cynical terms. Nesson's conclusion about the social function of doubt may or may not be true; I shall not pursue it further. What I want to ask is whether the unexpected conclusion he draws arises from the moral imperative that we should not convict someone who might be innocent on a probabilistic basis, or from mathematical difficulties.

Contradictions occur whether the jury convicts all 25 prisoners, 24, or none. If the jury convicts the first prisoner in the dock on a 0.96 probability of his guilt, it must do so with all the remaining prisoners. However, that is equivalent to announcing that 25 men killed the guard, which we know to be false. If none of the prisoners is convicted, 24 guilty men go free. The only way in which the jury could obtain the statistically correct result for the group as a whole would be to acquit one man chosen at random; yet convicting 24 men chosen at random is also abhorrent.

Here is where the distinction between ethical paradox and mathematical error comes in. It looks as if we can solve the mathematical problem by convicting 24 prisoners chosen at random, but no one would assert that this solution would solve the ethical problem. If the jury took that line, they would be transgressing against the basic Anglo-American legal principle of judging each case on its merits, without predetermining guilt: 'innocent until proven guilty'. What the jury decides about case 25 would be determined in advance by whether it chose to locate the one 'not guilty' verdict among the first 24 cases. Of course, there is no guarantee that the man chosen for acquittal would actually be innocent: indeed, there is a 0.96 probability of his being guilty. In that sense, the ethically wrong thing to do would not even have solved the mathematical problem. It would produce the statistically correct result for the group, but not for any individual.

Whether the jury would be to blame if it reached 24 guilty verdicts arbitrarily has nothing to do with the level of potential loss in this case. The jurors would still have acted wrongly whether or not the death penalty was in force. This is a case about probabilities and their paradoxes, not about utilities. To convict, the jurors should be able to assert that they were incapable of being surprised by a wrong result, that they had no reasonable doubts that this particular man was one of the 24 guilty ones. Yet they know that, for each man, they stand a 0.04 chance of being *wrong*, and that for the entire group they stand only a 0.04 chance of getting the distribution of guilt and innocence *right*. It has been said that probability judgements would be an appropriate tool 'for any legal system that aimed solely to discover the truth more often than not',[16] but not for one that aims to dispense justice to individuals. However, a 0.04 chance of getting the distribution right for the group hardly makes it likely that even that minimal criterion will be satisfied.

If we want to maintain a strict *a priori* legal principle such as 'innocent until proven guilty', we will simply have to ignore probabilities altogether in this case. This limitation will affect our responsibility as moral agents: we will be responsible for not infringing upon the presumption of innocence, but we will not be responsible for getting the outcome right in terms of identifying the one innocent man and convicting the others. *In fact, we will have to accept that the rightness or wrongness of the jury's decision cannot depend on how things turn out – on outcome luck*. What is true in this case will be true much more generally in medical ethics, as I shall argue in the applied chapters of the book.

This case illustrates two problems for a utilitarianism based on probable consequences. First, even indubitably accurate probabilities entail statistical problems of the sort highlighted: the extreme unlikeliness of getting it right for the group and the individual simultaneously. Second, getting it right for the group has to be balanced against another, indisputably *ethical* value: not wishing to convict individuals solely on a probabilistic basis, if that means trespassing on the presumption of innocence.

Possibly a committed consequentalialist would reply that there is nothing particularly special about the presumption of innocence, any more than any other *a priori* principle. That would be a coherent objection, in that the principles 'beyond a reasonable doubt' and 'innocent until proven guilty' come out of somebody else's toolkit, as all *a priori* principles do for utilitarians (except, of course, the principle of maximizing utility). They are not instruments which utilitarians are obliged to use unless they can be shown to enhance overall utility. Yet that would be a very extreme reading which would step outside the established parameters of the case and the actual ethos of the courtroom – when utilitarianism prides itself on its realism.

It might be objected, perhaps by rule-utilitarians, that following an *a priori* principle such as 'beyond a reasonable doubt' in criminal prosecutions does in fact increase general utility in society. Even if in particular instances it leads to paradoxes of probability, it is better overall to follow that rule, because the principle minimizes wrongful convictions, or increases trust in the judicial system, or allows us to view our society as a civilized one in a way that tickles our collective ego. Even though the moral mathematics does not sum up, it might still be rational to believe that the probable outcome – acquittal of all 25 men – is the right outcome.[17]

More broadly, for someone like Robert Nozick this is true of any principle, so that principles have no independent validity: they are merely 'transmission devices for probability and for utility'.[18] That is, the validity of adopting any principle rests on decision-theoretic analysis, just as does the value of any possible choice or contemplated action: 'a justification of a principle P is a decision-theoretic structure, with the principle P occupying the place of an action, competing with specific alternatives, having certain probabilities of reaching certain goals with certain desirabilities, and so on.'[19] Principles are merely instrumental: their function is to increase overall utility, to maximize our chances of achieving our desires, and they are adopted or rejected purely on a decision-theoretic basis.[20]

The question would then become an empirical one: on the balance of probabilities, presumably, is it better for society to maintain that the balance of probabilities is not the best standard in a criminal action? Clearly this leads to infinite regress, not just in this instance, but also in the larger sense that moral luck undermines any consequentialism of actual outcomes. To justify the adoption of a general principle for society as a whole, presumably the actual outcome must be beneficial, but we have already seen that a consequentialism of actual outcomes cannot escape the paradoxes of moral luck. Furthermore, there is a circularity in relying on the values arrived at through decision-theoretical analysis in order to ratify the values arrived at through decision-theoretic analysis. Nozick himself can escape from circularity only by having recourse to the largely discredited arguments of sociobiology, speculating that we are wired by evolution to serve particular ends, and that those ends are what general utility should serve.[21]

Some utilitarians have talked as if having a better set of probability estimates, a better theory of probability, or a better set of techniques for calibrating probabilities could eliminate all paradox and establish utilitarianism firmly as the only possible answer. As Helga Kuhse and Peter Singer remark:

> The utilitarian view is striking in many ways. It puts forward a single principle that it claims can provide the right answer to all ethical dilemmas, if only we can predict what the consequences of our answers will be. It takes ethics out of the mysterious realm of duties and rules, and bases ethical decisions on something that almost everyone understands and values. Moreover, utilitarianism's single principle is applied universally, without fear or favour.[22]

In a similar vein, J. J. C. Smart writes:

> What utilitarianism badly needs, in order to make its theoretical foundations secure, is some method according to which numerical probabilities, even approximate ones, could in theory, though not always in practice, be assigned to any imagined future event...I do not know how to do this, but I suspect, from the work that is at present being done on decision-making, that the situation may not be hopeless.[23]

The problem is conceived as admitting of a 'technical fix', but the example of the 25 prisoners shows that, no matter how indubitable the probabilities, paradox cannot be eliminated. If this is so, then Bentham's hopes in utilitarianism were misplaced, particularly insofar as method was meant to be a bulwark against luck: 'Every circumstance by which the condition of an individual can be influenced, being remarked and inventoried, nothing...[is] left to chance, caprice, or unguided discretion, everything being surveyed and set down in dimension, number, weight and measure.'[24]

Let us recapitulate the argument of this chapter so far. It seemed at first that consequentialism, in particular utilitarianism, could avoid the dilemma of moral luck because it emphasizes outcomes rather than the good will. However, consequentialists have been unable to agree on whether actual or potential outcomes are the standard by which to judge actions. There are serious reasons to doubt whether reliance on actual consequences avoids the paradox of moral luck, because actual consequences are typically outside moral agents' full control or predictive ability. When this is true, a consequentialism of actual consequences, like Brandt's, becomes harsh and obsessive in its counsels of perfection.

This difficulty, along with the related moral luck question of what agents can then be considered responsible for, if not outcomes, is adduced by Russell as grounds for emphasis on potential consequences instead – probabilities. Using potential or probable consequences as the touchstone appears to allow us recourse to statistical analyses of how similar events typically turn out (e.g., in evidence-based medicine). They also offer a less perfectionist standard for clinicians, who are then responsible for getting it right in the long run: attaining clinical standards over all their cases that fall within, say, one standard deviation of the normal outcomes for that particular procedure. But while probabilities may be a source of some enlightenment, they cannot do everything that has been claimed for them by such utilitarians as Smart.

In particular, no amount of improvement in the accuracy of probabilities can abolish conflicts in incommensurable values. Of course, in the case of the 25 prisoners, we would like to get the outcome right in the sense of apportioning acquittal and punishment correctly, but our prior value is not to convict an innocent man. In this case it seemed that the only solution was not to hold the jurors responsible for matching their verdicts to the probability distribution – convicting 24 men chosen at random, in conformity with the probability of 0.96

for each man being guilty. Only by not making the jurors responsible for getting the mathematically correct outcome could we avoid being intolerably surprised by how the outcomes turn out if the innocent man is convicted. Only by limiting what the jurors are responsible for – to upholding the legal principles of 'beyond a reasonable doubt' and 'innocent until proven guilty' – is it possible to avoid the paradox of moral luck. In this case, the jurors must *deliberately ignore* probable outcomes in order to do the ethically right thing and so escape moral luck.

Remorse and regret

There remains one set of questions about ill-luck in outcomes that has been suggested by this chapter but not yet fully considered: how badly the conscientious agent should feel if things turn out wrong. I began by suggesting that consequentialism looks at first as if it can avoid the problem of moral luck, because it shifts our concern from the character of the agent (as in virtue theory) or the purity of the good will (as in Kantianism) to the beneficial or adverse outcome of the action. The argument in the rest of the chapter has sought to demonstrate that this is not so, and that consequentialism cannot escape the paradoxes of moral luck. If that is true, then our concerns about the purity of the good will or the character of the agent resurface. In this final section, I want to discuss them at somewhat greater length, beginning with the instance of the conscientious health care professional but introducing broader concerns about agents' remorse and regret.

Let us return to Brandt's example of the consumer who should be able to avoid bad decisions by being adequately informed, and let us contrast that comparatively ideal situation with the usual situation in medicine. Evidence-based medicine can be seen as an 'attempt to avoid all mistakes deriving from inadequate reflection' by providing a better database through randomized clinical trials and meta-analyses. Yet even the most completely researched data will always be probabilistic, and statistical independence means that the case before this doctor, now, may well be the equivalent of the aberrant 'lemon'. How should the conscientious doctor react if she makes the wrong diagnosis, undertakes a procedure that turns out to have serious side effects or prescribes the wrong treatment, despite having conscientiously researched all the information? Assuming that there is no medical negligence involved in the actual performance of the procedure or diagnosis, presumably the doctor would view herself as justified 'in the long run', not by the outcome of this particular case. That is, assuming that in the long run the doctor's own results roughly approximate to the data gathered from statistical meta-analyses, she could view herself as having acted correctly even if one particular case turns out badly. This is indeed the basis of disciplinary proceedings against allegedly incompetent doctors, and a competent doctor, such as Wendy Savage, can survive such proceedings by showing that her results are as good or better than the average, even if particular cases turn out badly. By contrast, the Kennedy inquiry of July 2001 into the doctors in the Bristol paediatric heart surgery cases involved extensive comparisons with results obtained by other hospitals and other surgeons. The Bristol surgeons were not blamed for 'getting it wrong' in one case, but for getting it badly wrong over the long run. In medicine it seems clear that it is probable consequences and statistical aggregates that matter most. But that does not entirely eliminate the question of how the doctor should feel about the individual case that turns out badly. In the case of the Bristol babies, the parents' constant complaint was that the two principal surgeons showed no regret or remorse, much as in the case of the Alder Hey pathologist that I touched on in chapter 2.

What precisely is the content of the doctor's duty? The doctor has a duty of care towards each patient as an individual. This duty is arguably similar to that of the conscientious juror, which is to each individual accused person and not towards a statistical aggregate. In the Nesson example, we saw that the conscientious juror is in fact required to put aside the figures for the 25 prisoners as a whole, which would dictate choosing one prisoner at random to be acquitted, and concentrate on getting it right in each individual case. Getting it right meant acting according to two *a priori* principles, 'beyond a reasonable doubt' as the standard of proof in criminal cases, and 'innocent until proven guilty'. Each man was being tried on his own, and each deserved to have his case kept separate from any considerations about the aggregate, if we wanted to maintain basic legal principles. We had to get each trial right in light of those principles. Getting it wrong would have included the case in which the jurors consciously decide to let the twenty-fifth man go, having found against the previous 24, for no other reason than that this *was* the twenty-fifth man, and that they were anxious to get the overall distribution statistically correct. The importance of getting it right had nothing to do with whether the death penalty was in force; similarly, getting it right in medical ethics is just as important in chronic care as in acute care, in everyday matters as in life-and-death cases.

The effect of concentrating on these prior principles is to relieve much of the stress inherent in the duties of a juror, or a doctor. The juror or doctor is not necessarily responsible for getting the outcome right – rather, for following the right procedure. In the Nesson example, that procedure was based on long-established legal principles. In the next six chapters, I shall consider areas of medical ethics where we generally have no such precedents, and where the right procedure is not so easy to determine. In some areas, however, such as informed consent, we do have substantial guidance.

Nevertheless, it would be unreasonable to expect the jurors in Nesson's case (or cases) to go away feeling light-hearted and free, when a guard has died and no one has been convicted for his murder. Similarly, although the duties of the doctor are to the individual patient, it would be unreasonable for the doctor herself not to think about her overall record, not least in light of the increasing emphasis from outside sources on audit, clinical governance and league tables. What is difficult to delineate is how badly the agent should feel when the right procedures are followed but the outcome still turns out badly.

We seem to want agents like doctors, acting as moral agents, to be able to feel something like regret or even remorse, a much stronger emotion that does not normally apply in ordinary prudential decisions. When I discover that my new car has turned out to be a 'lemon' even though I followed rational decision procedures such as perusing *Consumer Reports*, I may well feel, regretfully, that 'I could kick myself', but I would hardly expect to feel guilty or remorseful. Yet if I am a paediatric heart surgeon, even one with an exemplary record in difficult procedures, I should probably feel something more than 'I could kick myself' when a baby dies during a procedure that I am performing. What exactly should that be? Remorse seems too strong, but regret seems too weak.

Bernard Williams introduces an alternative to regret and remorse: 'agent-regret', which is connected to failure not only of the agent's 'project' but, more fundamentally, to his own failure. Agent-regret is felt specifically about the agent's past actions, rather than about external states that have gone wrong. That is, the agent is not divorcing himself from the success or failure of his project. Its success may or may not be his, but the actions that he took to set it in train certainly are. To return to the example of Gauguin, 'what would prove him wrong in his project would not just be that it failed, but that he failed.'[25] Gauguin's self-identity is so intimately bound up in his art that the miscarriage of his artistic ambitions would have meant not only that his decision to abandon his commitments in France for Tahiti was wrong, but also that he himself was evil, to put the argument in a deliberately forceful fashion. I do not now want to discuss the difficult points about hindsight and moral luck that I have rehearsed elsewhere, particularly in chapter 1. The point I wish to resurrect here is the tightness of the link between Gauguin's profession and his sense of his own agency and worth.

Clearly there is a parallel with health professionals here. 'Getting it wrong' is something more than just 'project failure' or 'ill-luck in outcomes' in the health professions, and Nozick's language of maximizing preferences is utterly alien. The duty of care that the doctor or nurse owes to each individual patient forbids the health professional to write off a 'failure' in such comforting terms as 'better luck next time'. This is the source of remorse: the combination of a lowered sense of one's professional self-esteem and failure to provide the best standard of care.

But there is also a difference, and one that makes agent-regret less useful in health care ethics than Williams finds it in the Gauguin example. The health care professional owes a duty of care, enforced by the professional bodies and the law, to the patient; it is hard to see how Gauguin owes a 'duty to his art', except as a cliché. Therefore it is less useful to separate the outcomes for the patient of the health professional's actions from the acts themselves. What affects the patient is the outcome, not the intention or the action of the professional. Yet what the paradox of moral luck highlights is the imperfect control that agents possess over outcomes. So we seem to be back to the same difficulty again: given the paradox of moral luck, how much remorse or regret can we expect the conscientious doctor or nurse to feel about outcomes where control is not entirely assured, and the outcome turns out wrong?

A health professional cannot be expected to drag herself through agonies of remorse each time the statistically inevitable occurs, when the one patient in 100 with a potentially fatal condition dies under a course of treatment having a 0.99 probability of curing that condition. Nor would we expect the doctor to forgo that course of treatment for future patients, assuming no better odds can be obtained from new developments. Indeed, if 0.99 is the best rate of success available from all the alternative treatments, a consequentialist, at least, would claim that the doctor was at fault if she did *not* prescribe that course. Proponents of evidence-based medicine would also probably say so.[26]

Perhaps in such cases all we can ask the health care professional to feel, after all, is ordinary regret. As Williams himself notes,

> Regret necessarily involves a wish that things had been otherwise, for instance that one had not had to act as one did. But it does not necessarily involve the wish, all things taken together, that one had acted otherwise.[27]

And further,

> While [the agent's] justification is in some ways a matter of luck, it is not equally a matter of all kinds of luck. It matters how intrinsic the cause of failure is to the project itself.[28]

It also matters how intrinsic the duty to 'get it right this time' is to one's professional sense of worth. Thus health care administrators and political decision-makers, who are responsible for the overall allocation of resources, may not be bound by as strict a duty of care as medical professionals. Yet we would still want to say that they should carry some portion of blame if things turn out badly. In the Bristol inquiry, for example, it was noted that the level of staffing for children's heart surgery was suboptimal, that children were placed alongside adults in a mixed intensive care unit, and that paediatric cardiac surgery was 'tacked on' to the adult service.[29] The blame for the appallingly bad outcomes was not the surgeons' alone, insofar as resource allocation on the 'macro' or 'meso' levels was not their decision: they could decide only on the 'micro' level of each individual patient. (Issues concerning moral luck in resource allocation will be dealt with in chapter 6.)

In much of medical practice, the compelling cases are those involving mixed feelings: standing by a 'rational' decision that turned out badly, or ruing a lucky but ill-made one. Yet this is true not only of medical practice, but of life in general. The cases introduced in chapter 1, such as Nagel's example of the lorry driver who swerves to avoid the pedestrian, pertain more widely. The first three chapters of this book have established the centrality of the moral luck paradox, its imperviousness to a utilitarian solution, and its universality. The paradox of moral luck does not arise just by asking Kantian questions, nor is it only a problem for a Kantian, I have argued. In the next six chapters I want to show how widely the problem of moral luck does pertain in medicine, in areas from genetic screening to resource allocation. I also want to offer some possible precepts for lessening the problem. Risk, uncertainty, evidence-based reasoning and a range of other related concepts play major roles in these chapters, too. I begin in chapter 4 with what is perhaps the most generic topic, informed consent to treatment.

4

Risk and Consent

Consent to treatment is a promising area in which to begin exploring the practical implications of moral luck for medical ethics – along with the associated concerns of risk analysis, uncertainty and rationality. In broad terms, I have been asking whether the concepts of 'luck' and 'moral' are incompatible: whether or not there is a purely ethical realm unaffected by the uncertainty of outcomes, whether risk undermines ethics. The first question to ask about informed consent in medical ethics, then, is whether it eliminates questions about risks. If a patient gives her consent to a medical procedure, is the doctor free from moral blame if the procedure turns out badly?

Clearly this is a question about moral luck, and it will be the main one in this chapter. But some people will think it is an odd question. They see consent as a legal requirement, having nothing to do with 'moral blame' or, for that matter, 'moral praise'. Someone would not be praised for getting a consent; it just has to be done, to satisfy legal requirements and to avoid the tort of battery. If there is a moral question about responsibility, the law pre-empts it, in this view. Perhaps the question is not so much whether informed consent transfers responsibility to the patient, but rather whether it conceptualizes responsibility as having obeyed the law. If the doctor has obtained an informed consent, by this argument, that is the end of the matter: she has fulfilled the legal requirement and can take refuge in having done so. If not, she is responsible for having failed to obey the law, regardless of whether or not the procedure turns out well.[1]

I want to argue something different and, I hope, rather more subtle. In my view it is the giving of informed consent that stops the probability machine rolling, and that shuts out questions about moral luck and risk for the doctor. If the patient has given her informed consent

to treatment, both ethical and legal requirements have been fulfilled, provided always that the procedure is not performed negligently.
Through sheer statistical necessity, however, some outcomes will be
unfavourable even if performed non-negligently. The question raised
by moral luck considerations is who bears responsibility for those
outcomes. I want to argue that what informed consent does, if properly obtained, is to transfer responsibility for ill-luck in outcomes
from doctor to patient.

No matter how badly the procedure turns out, there is no cause for
remorse in the doctor who has obtained a properly informed consent,
although of course there will be grounds for regret. If the procedure
goes badly this particular time, the doctor will still be exempt from
either legal responsibility or ethical blame so long as she has obtained
informed consent from the patient beforehand.[2] The particular outcome will be a project failure rather than a personal failure for her,
and moral luck will not have undermined her agency. Nor will she
have neglected the duty of care that she owes to each patient as an
individual – which forbids her to write off a failure as a matter of
'better luck next time'. That duty will have been met through
obtained informed consent, although of course the doctor will still
be bound by the normal standards of medical negligence in the
performance of the procedure. Conversely, if the doctor fails to obtain
informed consent, and fails to disclose relevant risks to the patient,
she is to blame even if the procedure turns out well.

The law of consent: prudent patient versus reasonable doctor

It will be clear that this is a deontological rather than a consequentialist position. Such is the tenor of the law, too, particularly US law
relevant to informed consent:

> Every human being of adult years and sound mind has a right to
> determine what shall be done with his own body.[3]

> Anglo-American law starts with the premise of thorough-going self-
> determination. It follows that each man is considered to be master of
> his body, and he may, if he be of sound mind, expressly prohibit the
> performance of life-saving surgery, or other medical treatment. A doctor
> might well believe that an operation or form of treatment is desirable or
> necessary, but the law does not permit him to substitute his own judge-
> ment for that of the patient by any form of artifice or deception.[4]

Respect for the patient's right to self-determination on particular therapy demands a standard set by law rather than one which physicians may or may not impose on themselves.[5]

Every patient...shall be provided by the physician [with] the right to informed consent [and]...in the case of a patient suffering from any form of breast cancer, to complete information on all alternative treatments [to mastectomy] which are medically viable.[6]

The irony, of course, is that generally the law is brought into play only if the procedure turns out badly.[7] In this respect the law may be said to be consequentialist; but how else could a patient obtain standing to sue? The fact that the operation or treatment ended disastrously is not sufficient proof of failure to obtain consent, of course, since negligence may be involved. (However, an unhappy outcome is also insufficient proof of negligence: it must also be shown that the negligence caused the injury directly, and that the doctor was operating at a level of competence below the average for her profession.) Nevertheless, outcome ill-luck is usually a necessary practical requirement for launching a lawsuit. In this sense the doctor does not need that protection which informed consent offers – by transferring responsibility to the patient – when outcome luck is favourable.

There are exceptions, at least where professional disciplinary proceedings are concerned. A district health authority attempted unsuccessfully to discipline the consultant obstetrician Wendy Savage on grounds of professional incompetence in five cases. Three of these had actually turned out favourably. When Dr Savage argued that these cases had clearly been dredged up, by trawling through files, by opponents of her patient-centred style, the opposing barrister retorted, 'That is also the answer of the driver who rounds a blind corner on the wrong side of the road.' However, the inquiry subsequently found for Dr Savage, apparently on the grounds that her average level of competence was actually above that of her colleagues, who were not being disciplined. The issue of outcome luck was not the crux of the finding.

When the outcome is unfavourable, the remedies available in American and English law differ fundamentally, although perhaps less fundamentally than they did a decade ago.[8] The American case law on consent attempts to exclude moral luck by requiring *all* risks to be disclosed, very broadly speaking.[9] In contrast, English law tries to eliminate the paradoxes of probability and the vagaries of moral luck by not requiring that the patient be informed of *any* risks. American law concentrates on the rights of 'consumers', English law on the duties of providers. Although Lord Scarman argued for a 'prudent/reasonable patient' standard in his dissenting opinion in *Sidaway*, the majority opinion used a 'reasonable doctor' standard instead. The 'prudent patient' standard is similar to that prevailing in American and Canadian law, but the 'reasonable doctor' remains the English touchstone.[10] Why are the two approaches so disparate?

American populism versus English elitism may well be part of the answer,[11] but another component is the tension between 'informed' and 'consent'. I suggested earlier that the patient's consent does at first appear to make the morality of treatment risk-free for the doctor, to absolve her of blame and liberate her from remorse if the procedure turns out badly. 'Consent' seems to get rid of risk. But the consent must be *informed*, and that means telling the patient about the risks. These two components of informed consent pull in different directions, as reflected in the discrepancy between American and English law.

A well-known example of the more rights-centred and patient-orientated approach to consent in American case law is the California case of *Cobbs* v. *Grant* (1972), in which the court found that a surgeon, Grant, had failed to disclose a chain of low-probability risks to an ulcer patient, Cobbs. The overwhelmingly unlikely simultaneous occurrence of all these adverse events – injuries to the spleen, development of a new gastric ulcer and premature absorption of sutures – catapulted the patient into hospital three more times, requiring the removal of his spleen and half of his stomach. Cobbs's general practitioner had discussed with him the risks inherent in general anaesthesia, and Dr Grant had explained the nature of the operation. In court Grant's lawyer argued that it was not normal medical practice to divulge any more than this – relying on the same sort of argument that underpins English law on consent. But the court rejected doctor-centred modes of argumentation, refusing to accept that the question was how doctors defined their duties rather than how patients construe their rights. Noting that 'the patient's right of self-decision is the measure of the physician's duty to reveal', the court insisted that the surgeon should have disclosed 'all information relevant to a meaningful decision process'. This very wide construction of 'informed' raises all sorts of problems about decision-making under conditions of uncertainty. Before going on to examine them, it might be instructive briefly to compare the approach in English law.

Thirteen years after the *Cobbs* case, the highest English court upheld the argument rejected by the Californian justices – that it is entirely up to the doctor, or at least to the medical profession as a whole, to decide how much information the patient requires. Even if a doctor fails to disclose a serious risk in treatment, the patient's consent is still valid, according to the majority opinion in *Sidaway* v. *Board of Governors of Bethlem Royal Hospital* (1985). A patient who alleged that she would not have given her permission for elective surgery if she had been told all the risks was alleged to have given consent regardless. The High Court, Court of Appeal and House of Lords all disallowed the patient's claim for damages of £67,000, for severe disability following an operation on her cervical spine to relieve pain. Mrs Sidaway denied that the surgeon – whom she described as a 'man of very, very few words' – had revealed any possible side effects or risks of the operation to her, or indeed that he had informed her that the procedure was optional. Between the operation in 1974 and the final Law Lords judgment in 1985, the neurosurgeon had died. In stunningly circular fashion, the courts chose to assume that he had followed standard practice: to inform the patient of possible risk of damage to the nerve roots (the probability of which $= 0.02$) but not of possible damage to the spinal cord (where the probability $= 0.01$). It was the latter – with half the likelihood but a much greater loss, partial paralysis – that occurred in the case of Mrs Sidaway.

Now there are reasons to do with 'hindsight bias' that might make one sceptical of Mrs Sidaway's claim. 'Hindsight bias' describes the common tendency for people to claim in retrospect that they had much more certain knowledge of future outcomes at the time when they were making a decision than they actually possessed, according to contemporaneous measurements. For example, subjects asked to assess the chances of two sides in a battle where one side is apparently the underdog might assign a probability of success for the weaker side of 0.20, but subsequently claim they had given odds of 50–50 when told that the underdogs had in fact won. Hindsight bias might well make one doubt whether Mrs Sidaway was claiming to be more certain than she actually was at the time that she would not have consented to the procedure if she had known of the risk of paralysis. But this was not the basis for the Law Lords' decision.

To the extent that there is a body of English law on informed consent, it is intimately linked to the law of medical negligence, and in particular to the *Bolam* criterion used since 1957 in negligence actions.[12] In *Bolam* it was held that 'a doctor is not guilty of negligence if he has acted in accordance with a practice accepted as proper by a responsible body of medical men skilled in that particular act.'[13] However satisfactory or unsatisfactory this criterion may be in the negligence context, as Brazier and Miola argue, 'what is much more disturbing is that the *Bolam* test has been allowed to become the litmus test not just of clinical practice but of medical ethics... [In particular] "informed consent" was hustled into a *Bolam* straitjacket.'[14] In terms relevant to this book, a separate corpus of jurisprudence is logically required to deal with informed consent, where the risks are about what can go wrong 'normally', in the absence of negligent practice. But the judgment in *Sidaway* allows doctors to be judge and jury in their own cases where either negligence or consent is concerned.[15]

Even more recent English cases, such as the Court of Appeal judgment in *Bolitho* (1998), still tend more towards the 'reasonable doctor' standard in assessing risks than the 'prudent patient' one. Although Dillon LJ insisted that doctors' decisions were not exempt from judicial scrutiny, he held that, in order to question the defendant's evidence of support for his practice from a 'responsible body of medical men', a court overruling that evidence must be 'clearly satisfied that the views of that group of doctors were... views such as no reasonable doctor could have held.' He continued, 'That would be an impossibly strong thing to say of the honest views of experts.'[16] Furthermore, Lord Browne-Wilkinson explicitly excluded 'questions of disclosure of risk'[17] from the situations in which doctors can properly be held liable in negligence.

None the less, there have been some recent English cases that suggest the courts are becoming more prepared to take a stricter line about what risks doctors must disclose. In *Smith* v. *Tunbridge Wells Health Authority*[18] the court held that failure to warn a young man of impotence as a possible side effect of rectal surgery deprived the patient of informed choice. In *Pearce* v. *United Bristol Healthcare NHS Trust*,[19] however, a woman whose baby was stillborn following the doctor's failure to warn her of the risks of stillbirth without a Caesarean section or induced delivery lost her action to prove that failure to advise her of that risk was negligent. Lord Woolf's judgment excuses the doctor on the basis that the 'very, very small additional risk' to the child was not a sufficiently 'significant' risk. As in *Sidaway*, where the smaller risk was by far the more serious, this judgment ignores the magnitude of the possible loss, considering only its probability. However, the judgment also suggests a departure from the 'reasonable doctor' standard: 'if there is a significant risk which would affect the judgment of a *reasonable patient*, then in the normal course it is the responsibility of a doctor to inform the patient of that significant risk, if the information is needed so that the patient can determine for him or herself as to what course she should adopt.'[20]

Remorse, responsibility and consent

The usual critique of allowing doctors to decide what risks they should tell their patients about is framed deontologically, in terms of autonomy and paternalism.[21] There are also consequentialist grounds for distrusting the 'professional standard' approach in *Sidaway*: it becomes the profession's interest to narrow the scope of 'normal' disclosure. A moral luck approach to consent would suggest that it is actually not in the doctor's own interest to wield so much apparent power as the *Sidaway* standard allows – not if she wants to avoid regret and remorse. This is not intended as a paternalistic argument against paternalism, nor is it about what the prudent course would be for the doctor. It is an expressly ethical question, hinging on the transfer of responsibility through informed consent.

After the Court of Appeal had found against Mrs Sidaway, the editor of the *Medico-Legal Journal* wrote:

> [In the court's view] it is a matter for the doctor to decide how much or how little he should tell his patient, taking into account all the circumstances of which he knows, including the patient's true wishes. As Sir John [Donaldson, Master of the Rolls, giving judgment] pointed out, though many patients may say they want to be told all, it is clear that some of them don't. It is for the doctor to divine which is the case . . . The doctor would seem to have to be a cross between a detective, a fortune teller, and an emotional and rational prop in some cases . . . The responsibility is heavy.[22]

Just so. Doctors might be expected to prefer telling their patients as much as possible, in order to absolve themselves of responsibility if the procedure misfires. Yet of a group of over 200 British doctors from hospital and general practice, 88 per cent asserted that they would not inform a patient if her cancer was likely to prove fatal. The remainder would generally inform patients whom they judged to be intelligent and emotionally stable; sometimes they would also inform lesser mortals. The majority of these doctors said they would tell a relative instead, although in English law relatives have no power to consent to treatment on behalf of an adult patient. Yet 60 per cent of these same doctors wanted to be told themselves if they had cancer.[23]

These survey results date from 1961, and there is evidence of a shift towards fuller disclosure since that more paternalistic period.[24] So long as English law allows doctors to take refuge in silence, however, there will still be a considerable number who tell the patient nothing: a full 33 per cent of general practitioners surveyed in Sheffield in 1986 still kept a terminal diagnosis from their patients.[25] Precisely nothing is what my husband and I were told when my mother-in-law died in a London hospital in September 1999. We were reduced to surreptitiously reading her bedside notes under cover of a newspaper: the diagnosis of advanced renal cancer was there, and there alone. As late as the day of her death we were refused a consultation with the senior registrar in charge of her case. On that same day a well-intentioned nursing sister suggested a syringe driver to palliate the pain, beginning her talk with us by saying, 'Of course you know what's wrong, the doctor will have told you.' But no one had told us anything.

The nursing sister came closest of anyone to telling us what was wrong with my mother-in-law, and perhaps this was no coincidence. Some commentators feel that nurses have a stronger commitment to truth-telling and disclosure than doctors do.[26] If this is true, perhaps it is because doctors typically have greater power and authority over patients; sharing information and knowledge with patients threatens that power.[27] (It is a truism that information is power, of course.) A substantial difference between the professions in their views on informed consent was illustrated by the motion passed by the British Medical Association's annual meeting in 1987, when doctors called for compulsory mass HIV screening of all patients on general practitioners' lists. The screening was to be done in secret, if need be – without specific informed consent for that procedure, even if general consent to taking blood for another purpose had been obtained. At the same time the nurses' central professional body, the United Kingdom Central Council on Nursing, Midwifery and Health Visiting, warned its members that nurses who co-operated in such screening would be liable to disciplinary measures. An interview with a sample of nurses found the majority opposed to testing for HIV without patients' explicit consent.[28] At their next annual meeting the doctors rescinded their 1987 motion, but it was unclear if their change of heart was due to their realizing the ethical implications about lack of informed consent, or to legal advice that they would be open to litigation.

Opacity has often been the order of the day in routine screening for HIV among all pregnant women presenting for antenatal care. Since 1990 anonymized unlinked screening had been official policy, primarily for epidemiological purposes. At the time the policy was instituted, treatment with antiretrovirals such as AZT was not yet available; thus it could be argued that little good would be done by telling women their diagnosis.[29] Now the situation is different, and the consequentialist arguments chime with the deontological ones. By abstaining from breastfeeding and undergoing treatment with antiretrovirals, women can reduce the risk of vertical transmission to the baby and their own risk as well. Yet the policy of non-disclosure continues – with objectors met with the retort that any woman who wishes can always obtain a separate test from a genito-urinary clinic, so that there is in fact full disclosure.[30] This seems to be a gross dereliction of responsibility.

Rationality and risk

The moral mathematics in *Sidaway* raise deeply problematic issues, and it is understandable, if not condonable, that English courts have tried to skirt them. Should patients be informed of all risks with a probability greater than 0.01? – the risk of partial paralysis, which Mrs Sidaway was not told about. Why not 0.02? – the likelihood of partial paralysis of the nerve ends, which Mrs Sidaway was warned of. How about 0.05? Any boundary will be arbitrary, particularly if the risk with the lesser probability carries the greater loss – as in Mrs Sidaway's case. Worse still, we cannot always know what the probabilities are before the disasters occur, especially with experimental treatments.

Advocates of evidence-based medicine will reply that it is precisely the function of EBM to ascertain the degrees of probability of success for various treatments with greater accuracy. If it were simply a matter of establishing those more accurate probabilities and presenting them to patients, in order that they can balance clinical probabilities and their own utilities more rationally, that would be laudable. However, there is ample evidence that EBM is also used as a rationing tool in order to deny patients treatments and services they want and need. Although multiple sclerosis patients have consistently demanded that beta-interferon should be available on the NHS, a long saga of preliminary and slightly less preliminary statements from the National Institute for Clinical Excellence culminated in August 2001 with the judgement that, based on evidence from clinical trials, the benefits of beta-interferon did not outweigh the cost of some £10,000 per patient per year.[31] Rightfully speaking, evidence-based medicine can establish only the probabilities of success or failure with a given treatment; the utilities attached to those probabilities are for individual patients to decide. Further, drug-based treatments for acute illness are the usual stuff of EBM; there will remain a large class of unexamined treatments – particularly in psychiatry and neonatal medicine, where clinical trials are ethically dubious or where consent from experimental subjects is difficult to obtain.[32]

Mrs Sidaway was in severe pain before the operation, even though the procedure was an elective one. If the pain is sufficiently great, is it irrational to accept a high level of risk? Borrowing the idea of identity from Bernard Williams[33] – although not the direction of his argument – might we ask whether a person in great pain is almost a different person from the 'same' person after the pain-relieving operation? If this is so, then the problem verges on the issue of what risks it is right for one person to impose on another. I will provide a more extended analysis of that question in chapters 7 and 8, drawing on examples from reproductive medicine and psychiatry; here I want to sketch out a preliminary account of what the problem is.[34]

There are two clear-cut alternative positions about whether others have the right to impose risk on us and, if so, what limitations there are to that right. On the one hand, it might be held that we have an absolute right against the imposition of risks by others without our consent. Although this position sounds like common sense, it is actually rather counter-intuitive: other people impose risks on us all the time, and it is hard to imagine how we could live without likewise imposing some risks on others. Besides, this position fails to distinguish between major and minor harms. Some rights infringements seem to carry too small a probability of harm to worry about. Thus Judith Jarvis Thomson, for example, prefers a 'high-risk' thesis: that we have rights only against others' attempts to impose major risks on us.[35] But, as we have seen in the *Sidaway* case, what counts as 'major' to the patient may be 'minor' to the doctor. In addition, some acts pose simultaneous small risks to a very large number of agents: pollution, for example.

On the other hand, one might take the position that it is perfectly permissible to impose risks on others, provided that compensation is offered. This position also leads to the counter-intuitive extremes of Robert Nozick's account,[36] in which there are no prohibitions on imposing risk if the right level of restitution is offered. Some harms are just not permissible to impose, no matter how unlikely. For example, playing Russian roulette on Jones without his consent with a bullet in one of a hypothetical million chambers is not the same as going for a drive in the country and thus imposing a one in a million risk on Jones if he steps out of his cottage door at the wrong time. Admitting that there are some risks which we can rightfully impose on others also makes us vulnerable to slippery slope problems: once we start quantifying the limits of the risks that it is acceptable to impose, we seem to be on very shaky ground. So there must be some other factor that makes imposing a risk impermissible, beyond probability and loss (balanced together against the pleasure I derive from the act, which is assumed to be equivalent in both cases). It sounds as if what that extra something might be is in fact malevolent intention, a Kantian notion that cannot be incorporated into a decision-theoretic, utilitarian analysis. The first action intends Jones's death in a more direct, malevolent way than the second – or at least derives pleasure from contemplating the possibility of Jones's death.

I have argued so far that the function of informed consent is to bypass both these counter-intuitive results for luck in outcomes, by allowing the patient to determine what risks are acceptable and to accept responsibility for how those risks turn out. Against that view, it might be argued that an absolutist notion of consent is as troublesome as an absolute notion of rights – equally impractical and counter-intuitive. We can't and don't seek the consent of everyone whom we expose to risk, even intentionally. This argument has been used to justify anonymity for seropositive doctors, or for doctors with hepatitis B. On this view, patients run all sorts of much more major risks in everyday life than they will encounter in visiting a doctor or dentist who has not declared to them his immunological status. Provided that the doctor takes reasonable precautions, there are no grounds for barring him from practice on the grounds of risk imposition on patients.[37]

This may be true in everyday life, but is it true in medicine? Does the duty of care make a crucial difference? I would argue that it does: there is a prior duty not to expose patients to risk – the underpinning concept in medicine of *primum non nocere*, first do no harm. The

doctor is specifically required not merely to lack a malevolent intention, but to intend benefit; where benefit is not possible, at the very
least the clinician should not harm the patient, and the beginning of
that particular wisdom is not imposing risk of harm. There are also
other differences between medicine and everyday life, where it is often
difficult to know who the potential risk bearers are. This is not true in
clinical medicine, where the issue is very precisely focused on a
particular treatment or procedure. (It may be more true in double-
blind randomized clinical trials, where we do not know until the trial
is over whether the control or the experimental group bore greater
level of risk; the trial begins from an assumption of equipoise, with no
prior beliefs about the effectiveness or riskiness of either treatment
arm.) Further, whereas it is difficult to obtain consent from all concerned in the everyday case of a low-level risk imposed on large
numbers of people, clinical medicine is typically about the one-
to-one encounter between doctor and patient. Finally, in some branches of medicine, particularly psychiatry, doctors can be held accountable not only for the risks they themselves impose, but also for not
preventing harm to others – for example, when their assessments of the
risk posed by a patient released into the community are too optimi-
stic.[38] All these considerations point to the need for a different account
for doctors than for the rest of us of what risks it is right to impose.

How much is the doctor responsible for?

I have argued that, because doctors owe a prior duty of care to their
patients, it is not good enough to say that they can no more help
imposing risks than the rest of us can in everyday life. If that is so,
however, it seems to lumber doctors with a very heavy responsibility.
In this final section I want to undertake some conservative surgery
myself: reducing the realm of the ethical to the obtaining of informed
consent itself. That, in my view, is what doctors are responsible for.
They should not subject patients to risks without consent, but they are
not responsible for ill-luck in outcomes if risks have been 'properly'
communicated. I want to leave the notion of 'properly' until later
chapters, where I hope that specific content from particular clinical
areas will help to illuminate what it might mean, although I also deal
briefly with the notion of 'material risks' at the end of this section.

  If doctors are responsible only for obtaining the consent itself – and
of course for performing the procedure in a non-negligent fashion –

that is consistent with the position on moral luck which I developed in the first three chapters. There, too, I proposed a route out of the crippling paradoxes of moral luck that depended on limiting what agents are responsible for, but enforcing that limited responsibility strictly. The same is true of informed consent to treatment. Even if the treatment turns out to have an unfavourable outcome, the doctor has not acted *unethically* as long as she has obtained informed consent. She may or may not have acted negligently or imprudently – not necessarily in law, if she has performed at the standard of the average competent practitioner (the *Bolam* test). Even an extra-competent practitioner cannot evade ill-luck in outcomes altogether, but practitioners cannot be held responsible for the statistically inevitable unlucky outcome which will occur one in 100 times for a procedure with a 99 per cent success rate. I assume that no better odds than 99–1 are available from other treatments. One proviso we might want to add – and this does come from the evidence-based medicine outlook – is that it is also incumbent on the practitioner to make sure that no better odds are available. However, if there is a treatment that offers better odds – and this does not come from the EBM movement, but rather from the core of my own argument – it must be acceptable to the patient.

But what about the countervailing duties of a doctor? Some doctors will argue, in consequentialist fashion, that they are under a moral obligation to administer the treatment with the highest probability of cure – that they are not entitled *not* to impose the risks associated with that method. This claim is weakest when used to defend non-disclosure to patients. Not informing patients of their prognosis is no more likely to lessen their anxiety than telling them;[39] several studies have also documented the way in which patients who understand their diagnosis, prognosis and treatment regime are more likely to be compliant with that regime and to achieve better rates of cure.[40] When people with Hodgkin's Disease (a cancer of the lymph glands) were provided with written materials about their condition and treatment, they had lower levels of depression, stress and anxiety.[41] A meta-analysis of the effects of full information on patients' compliance and therapeutic outcomes demonstrated that 100 per cent of studies involving patients on antibiotics showed that a better clinical outcome was achieved with fuller information, and that 66 per cent of studies also showed better adherence to the treatment regime.[42] Interestingly, this finding may suggest that something other than compliance explains the better clinical outcome – perhaps participating actively in one's own care.

The claim that patient outcomes will be superior if informed consent is bypassed may be more tenable in a few exceptional instances, but even there it remains debatable. Where an adult patient cannot give consent, no one else can, in English law; the question then becomes whether the doctor has an obligation to proceed in the patient's best interests. Treatment for the patient's mental disorder can be authorized without consent under section (3) of the Mental Health Act 1983, although it must be treatment for a mental disorder rather than a physical condition (s63). It has been argued that the purpose of compulsory, non-consensual treatment is to restore the patient's autonomy, so that she can then give an informed consent or refusal to further treatment.[43] Apart from the emergency situation, however, there is a terrible temptation to abuse here.[44] The most blatant instance of such abuse in recent years in English law has been the imposition of enforced Caesarean sections on women judged to be incompetent and/or suffering from a mental illness – even though a Caesarean section is clearly a physical procedure, rather than treatment for a mental illness.[45] In addition to the legal reasons to be sceptical about this claim, there are also philosophical ones. Overriding patient autonomy so as to confer autonomy makes the patient a means towards the end of her own autonomy.

Another sort of consequentialist reasoning tries to defend withholding information from the patient or administering a placebo outside of the clinical trial context on outcome-orientated grounds. In one case, therapists successfully overcame a patient's drug addiction by substituting a placebo for the drug, without the patient's knowledge. When eventually informed of what had occurred, the patient was angry at first but later came to judge the 'treatment' with a placebo as a success in his own terms. 'They'll thank you afterwards', this argument runs, and it can be extremely tempting to clinicians. As the clinicians in this case later wrote, 'We felt ethically obliged to use a treatment that had a high probability of success...To withhold the procedure may have protected some standards of openness, but may not have been in his [the patient's] best interests.'[46] But what if the procedure had failed, and the patient had discovered the deception? Wouldn't that have damaged the therapeutic relationship beyond repair? And unless treatment by placebo had a 100 per cent rate of success, how could the therapists have known in advance that it would work? In many of the enforced Caesarean cases, the women were conspicuously 'ungrateful' for an intervention which carried a higher risk of mortality and morbidity to themselves and the baby, particularly in cases where women had previously undergone a successful vaginal delivery.[47]

In this case the therapists were not actually imposing a procedure, but rather withholding a drug; the responsibility appears merely negative. In both cases, however, medical staff arguably had a positive obligation to obtain consent. A third case, again one in which the doctor argued that he was justified by results, illustrates the looking-glass-world position of claiming to have acted in the patient's best interests when the patient has actually died. It is a compelling case, however, since, in the doctor's experience, the rate of failure for the procedure was zero.

The case involves a hospital urologist who never warned patients that they might have a fatal reaction during urography because he thought it would do no good. The death of one of his patients left him unmoved in his conviction that he had acted for the ethical best:

> I have done 6000 to 8000 urograms in the past thirteen years and no one has ever had a fatal reaction. We have been doing urograms at this hospital for at least 25 years, and no one has ever had a fatal reaction ... Because the indications for urography were great and the chances for a reaction were remote, I am sure I would have convinced Mrs E ... to have the procedures. She would then have had the reaction and died, and the fact that I warned her would have done Mrs E ... absolutely no good.[48]

Williams suggests that the attempt to evade moral luck is so central to an ethical way of thinking that we may prefer to abandon the moral enterprise altogether if we cannot escape from moral luck. The radiographer is doing just that: denying that there is any ethical issue, since moral luck is inescapable here. How can he excuse his failure to obtain informed consent as having produced the best available outcome, when the patient has died? How can he be so certain that he would have 'convinced' Mrs E to have the procedure? (Indeed, his use of the term 'convinced' says little for his respect for patients' autonomy.) Perhaps, when apprised of the gladsome tidings that there had been no deaths in urography for twenty-five years in this hospital, Mrs E would have remarked that it might well be her turn. That reaction smacks of Gambler's Fallacy – the mistaken conviction that a long run of blacks at roulette say, changes the probability of red on the next turn – but in this case it would not necessarily have been irrational. What is irrational is to assume, as the clinician did, that because the risk was zero in his own experience, it was zero across the board.

The best outcome, in clinical terms, needs to include process as well. The right way of making the decision is important. Conversely, the aim is not to spare patients worry – which is impossible – but to allow them to 'worry intelligently'.[49] On the other hand, it is naïve to think that all risks can be communicated. If the doctrine of informed consent is construed as requiring all risks to be disclosed, it cannot satisfy the Kantian 'ought implies can' standard. The problem is less severe if the doctor's duty is not to impart information about all possible risks, but about all the risks she knows.[50] Provided that this does not become an excuse for failing to keep abreast of research, this refo.mulation should satisfy a deontologist.

The doctrine of therapeutic privilege is invoked by some consequentialists to deny that doctors should reveal all risks even if they could. Certainly doctors need to avoid the macho approach of forcing information on patients who genuinely do not want to know; that, too, is the patient's right. And it will not always be easy to ascertain how much patients want to know without telling them what they don't want to know. A sensitive doctor may be able to find a detour that leads to the right place, as Dr Robert Buckman, an oncologist, relates in this story:

> I have a very vivid memory of a patient with cancer of the ovary whom I first met several years ago. The letter from her doctor said, 'She simply will not allow me to tell her what is going on, and I am concerned that you may not be able to offer her treatment.' She was an exceptionally nervous woman and her first words to me were, 'If it's cancer, I don't want you to tell me.' I assured that I would not and asked about her fears of cancer. She told me of the deaths of five members of her family years ago, and the sufferings they had endured. Her main fears were of similar suffering. She thought that if she knew it was cancer all the fight would go out of her. We talked for about half an hour and I described the treatment in detail and mentioned the various support services that we could offer (including more conversations about her fears). When she heard about the treatment she recognised it as chemotherapy, and when I said it was, she smiled broadly (for the first time) and said, 'Oh well, I knew it was cancer anyway.' From that moment on, she relaxed and was able to tolerate the treatment and several ups and downs of her disease with considerable calm.[51]

What Buckman succeeded in doing here was responding to the individual patient's unique and individual reasons to fear cancer. In so doing he showed an implicit awareness of the two alternatives enunciated in an early US consent case, *Salgo* v. *Leland Stanford Jr. University Board of Trustees*:

> One is to explain to the patient every risk attendant upon any surgical procedure or operation, no matter how remote; this may well result in alarming a patient who is already unduly apprehensive and who as a result refuses to undertake surgery in which there is in fact minimum risk; it may also result in actually increasing the risks by reason of the physiological results of the apprehension itself. The other is to recognize that each patient presents a separate problem, that the patient's mental and emotional condition is important and in certain cases may be crucial, and that in discussing the element of risk a certain amount of discretion must be employed.[52]

This nuanced view is a very long way from the proposition that consent forms constitute an iatrogenic harm to the patient. That claim is all the more presumptuous when applied to subjects in non-therapeutic experiments, who by definition receive no countervailing medical benefits.[53] None the less, even Buckman's careful approach may fall prey to the assumption that patients want to know less than they really do. Much of the literature reveals a gap between the number of risks that doctors normally disclose and the extent of risk information that patients profess to desire. An American survey, for example, discovered that doctors said they usually disclosed five or six out of a possible sixteen relevant facts about the probabilities of adverse side effects from seizure medication, whereas patients wanted to know an average of thirteen or fourteen such facts.[54] In the supposedly more deferential UK, 63 per cent of a group of 262 patients seeing a specialist at an outpatient clinic felt that they had not been told enough during the consultation.[55] Are patients perhaps more rational – in Richard Brandt's most basic sense of requiring as much information as possible[56] – than doctors take them to be? It would be pleasant to think so, but other studies suggest that they fail to make fully rational use of information – to measure up to Brandt's second criterion for rationality, that is, the elimination of cognitive bias.[57]

Twenty men with a previous history of hospitalization for heart disease were informed, in a taped interview before their current surgery, of the risk of death during the procedure, possible complications, likely benefits, probability of overall success, and alternative treatments.[58] When interviewed again after the operation, only 25 per cent remembered that the possibility of death during surgery had ever been mentioned. A full 90 per cent had forgotten that less serious complications had also been discussed. Even when the interviewers reminded the subjects that these topics had been included, 58 per cent of subjects could not remember the probability of death that had been given, and 77 per cent failed to recall either the content or the probability of other complications. Patients were better able to remember the benefits that had been predicted from a successful operation – indicating contamination of their thought by 'motivational biases', wishful thinking. Each of the patients was unable to recall at least one important component of the interview, and sixteen out of twenty positively denied that certain major items had come up. Thirteen out of twenty fabricated facts. One patient maintained stoutly that he had been given no information at all: 'All he [the doctor] did was lift up my shirt, put a stethoscope on my heart, and that was it.' This patient had in fact been given half an hour of the surgeon's time, time which the surgeon might well feel he could have spent on other pressing clinical matters.

As if this was not sufficient proof of irrationality, all the patients thought they knew more than they did. 'They were frequently in error but never in doubt.'[59] The patient who achieved the poorest recall scores was adamant that he could call to mind every word of the interview. All these patients had been 'educated' by previous experience of hospitalization: none was an emergency admission, none lacked mental capacity. It is possible that the patients were better informed at the time they signed the consent proforma but forgot the information postoperatively – indeed, perhaps wanted to forget it once the procedure was successfully over. None the less, in the absence of preoperative tests of comprehension, we cannot know for sure.

There are two positive points to draw out of these apparently negative findings. The first is that all the patients survived, which is rather remarkable, given their advanced pathology. Perhaps this study is further proof of the tendency for better clinical outcomes to be associated with full disclosure of information, as noted earlier. The second is that it would be wrong – an instance of the naturalistic fallacy, the illicit shift from what is to what should be – to claim that, because people fail *in fact* to exhibit perfect understanding of information, there is no obligation *in ethics* to inform them.[60]

The dilemma of inefficient use of information, and therefore of the doctor's time in imparting that information, is more serious for a consequentialist. A deontologist might assert that the doctor's duty is to inform to the best of her ability, but that the doctor cannot ensure comprehension, no matter how diligently she tries to minimize the fear and denial that patients such as Buckman's naturally feel. I find this a plausible way of limiting further what doctors are responsible for. In any case, doctors are not necessarily much better equipped to explain probabilities and risks than patients are to understand them. Roger Higgs, a general practitioner and professor of general practice, believes that doctors have a 'restricted and inflexible understanding of scientific probability'.[61]

American law has attempted to bridge the gap between patients' expressed desire for full information and their unimpressive track record with the information they are given by developing a doctrine of 'material risks'. This is the requirement that, before obtaining informed consent, the doctor must 'explain the procedure to the patient . . . and warn him of any material risks of danger inherent in or collateral to the therapy',[62] not of *all* the risks. A material risk is defined elsewhere in US case law as one which 'a reasonable person, in what the physician knows or should know to be the patient's position, would be likely to attach significance to.'[63]

Courts on both sides of the Atlantic have attempted to apply some similar standard of reasonability of the decision to adult patients even when their competence is in doubt. To their credit, courts in the UK have not necessarily assumed that competence is always illustrated by agreeing with the doctor or with the judge's own assessment of risk, although that temptation is always present. Refusing treatment can easily be seen as proof of irrationality, when treatment is presumed to be in the patient's best interests.[64] Indeed, that argument was made concerning a sixteen-year-old English anorexic who was refusing transfer to a treatment centre where she might be force-fed.[65] However, in another case involving an adult patient with long-standing schizophrenic delusions in an English secure hospital, the court allowed expert testimony to the effect that other elderly patients with vascular problems often refused the proposed treatment for gangrene – amputation – even though their competence was not in doubt.[66]

In a more poignant case, an American woman with arteriosclerosis of the brain, who was alternately rational and confused, was hospitalized by order of a lower court, without her consent, in order to stop the wandering to which she was prone when confused.[67] The woman brought an appeal, with her lawyers maintaining that the burden should be on the lower court to suggest alternative treatments for her wandering. When ordered to reconsider by the court of appeal, the district court held that, in her lucid moments, the woman would have seen that the rational decision was hospitalization. The rational self would have elected to hospitalize the mad self, and itself as hostage. The woman was returned to the mental hospital, where she died.

These legal cases are suggestive, but ultimately the 'reasonable' person is a moral concept, not simply a factual or legal one. It functions as a 'stand-in' for patient autonomy, as does the presumption of competence in adult patients. To summarize the argument in this chapter, it seems to me that the paradoxes of probability, rationality and risk require us to err on the absolutist side in our interpretation of informed consent. The doctor's responsibility is not to get the outcome right in all cases; indeed, even an extreme consequentialist would be hard pressed to defend that position, since a certain proportion of cases will turn out 'wrong' even when the statistical distribution for the practitioner is 'right'. Here the normal standards of negligence apply: the doctor will not be found negligent if she performs at the level of average competence for a physician in her circumstances, which may well include overwork, fatigue and other harbingers of outcome ill-luck.

Of course, if the only doctor in town is habitually drunk during half his operations, and admits as much to me beforehand, I can hardly be said to have consented freely if I allow him to operate on me for a fatal condition, so as to have at least a 50–50 chance of survival. But one hopes that he is below the normal clinical standard, and that he would be liable for negligence even if I had given my consent. In effect, his negligence would have changed the probabilities: they would have become very much worse than those I could have expected. Another way of putting this point is to say that, although the giving of informed consent does transfer responsibility to the patient, the doctor is still subject to the normal professional standards.

If a procedure turns out badly, the normally competent physician cannot be held ethically at fault if she has obtained informed consent. To put the matter in deliberately oversimplified terms, she will be unlucky but not evil, and should experience regret but not guilt or remorse. The doctor's responsibility is not necessarily to get the outcome right, but to proceed in the correct fashion. Both the consequentialist and the paternalist, by contrast, seem to be required to regard the doctor as a wrongdoer if the procedure turns out badly.

Thus an absolutist interpretation of consent protects both doctor and patient: the doctor from moral luck, and the patient from invasion of autonomy.

5

Death and Dying

In chapter 4, on informed consent to treatment, I proposed a way out of the moral luck maze that depended on limiting strictly what doctors are responsible for, but enforcing that responsibility equally strictly. In this chapter I want to look at some issues around death and dying that call into question the strictness with which that responsibility should be enforced. Earlier I wrote that doctors 'should not subject patients to risks without consent, but . . . are not responsible for ill-luck in outcomes if risks have been properly communicated'. Thus I conceptualized informed consent as transferring responsibility for ill-luck in outcomes from doctor to patient, provided that patients have understood and accepted the level of risks in the procedure and its side effects.

But what about cases in which communication is difficult or impossible? Much can and has been done to limit the scope of such cases: for example, whereas it used to be thought that children and young people would more or less automatically fall into the group of patients with whom communication is impossible, the British Medical Association working party on children's consent to treatment, of which I was a member, has shown quite definitively that this is not so.[1] Similarly, the 1997 report of the Ethics Advisory Committee of the Royal College of Paediatrics and Child Health recommends giving dying children a considerable degree of autonomy in accepting or rejecting life-prolonging treatment.[2] Recent research suggests a functional test of cognitive and emotional maturity, rather than a strict age cut-off point: the achievement of a stable set of values is possible at a comparatively early age.[3] However, even if children and young people are increasingly thought capable of accepting or refusing treatment on the basis of informed consent, in the area of death and dying there will remain some other very hard cases indeed, for adults and children alike. In this chapter I use the case of Tony Bland, a young man at the cusp of adulthood who exemplifies many of those issues. I begin with a description of the case and the question of whether it is right to withdraw life-sustaining treatment from patients in Bland's condition. In the next section the principal question concerns luck in outcomes in decisions about withdrawing or withholding life-sustaining treatment, although I will also make brief references to luck in antecedent circumstances and luck in the decisions that have to be faced. Later in this chapter I will return to the questions about consent. There another form of luck will join luck in outcomes: luck in character.

Withdrawal of life-sustaining treatment and assisted suicide

In the 1993 case of Anthony Bland[4] the Law Lords were faced with the question of whether to allow doctors to discontinue nasogastric feeding of an eighteen-year-old man who had suffered severe cerebral injuries. Accepting the diagnosis of Bland's condition as persistent vegetative state, Lord Keith described his situation as the rare one in which there is no medical uncertainty, but rather the terrible certainty of hopelessness:

> Anthony Bland cannot see, hear or feel anything. He cannot communicate in any way. The consciousness which is the essential feature of individual personality has departed forever.[5]

However, in 1996 a consultant in neurodisability and his colleagues published a disturbing paper in the *British Medical Journal* that cast doubt on how 'forever' is 'forever'. Of some forty patients diagnosed as being in persistent vegetative state and studied by Keith Andrews and his team at his specialist unit, 75 per cent had developed some further signs of consciousness, with some even being able to spell to command and do mental arithmetic communicating by eye, painting or touch-sensitive buzzer.[6] The findings of Andrews et al. must be troubling for the *Bland* case and subsequent jurisprudence founded upon it.[7] That supposed rare instance of medical certainty, persistent vegetative state, appears to be sliding back into the more typical morass of uncertainty, risk and luck. If it was not absolutely certain that Tony Bland's higher cerebral functions were permanently extinguished, would it still have been right to withhold life-sustaining treatment from him? If there was any vestige of hope, however slim, would accepting his death still have been the only option?

This is a particularly poignant case of ill-luck in outcomes. If doctors decide to maintain a patient diagnosed as being in a persistent vegetative state, on the admittedly slim hope of some recovery in higher brain function, one set of unhappy outcomes are all too probable: those of what is often termed a 'living death'. In the parallel case of Nancy Cruzan,[8] a 33-year-old American woman injured in a car accident who was fed artificially for seven years after being diagnosed in persistent vegetative state, the patient's family found her continued twilight existence unspeakably painful. Her body had atrophied so severely that her fingernails cut into her wrists. Like Tony Bland, she was able to follow movement with her eyes, in a cruel simulation of entering into relationship with family and friends, but this reflex action connoted nothing at all about her higher brain functions. In such cases, families are unable to grieve properly, and helpless to help: by taking her case to the Supreme Court, the Cruzan family were doing 'the only thing we can do, [that is] . . . to help her die.'[9]

But if doctors decide to withdraw life-sustaining treatment, including nutrition and hydration, from a patient in persistent vegetative state, they may be responsible for another kind of bad outcome: the death not of a patient who has no hope, but of the patient who could have recovered some degree of brain function, even if against the odds. That doctors can be held responsible for failing to treat someone to whom they have a duty of care, with the intention of allowing to die, is clear in criminal law.[10] So it is no good saying that the condition rather than the doctor kills the patient in this instance. It is true that the doctor does not actually kill the patient by administering lethal drugs, as in euthanasia, but the doctor still retains a measure of responsibility for the patient's death. Patients in persistent vegetative state may survive up to thirty years with parenteral or nasogastric nutrition and hydration. If nutrition and hydration is taken away from a patient to whom the doctor has a duty of care, it is withdrawing nutrition and hydration that results in the patient's death. That does not automatically mean that it is ethically wrong, or legally culpable, according to the *Bland* judgment; but the *Bland* judgment relies heavily on the supposedly absolute certainty that higher brain functions will never be regained.

It looks very much as if the doctors' responsibility, in decisions involving withdrawal of care more broadly, depends on how things turn out; but of course by pre-empting the decision to withhold nutrition and hydration, the doctors are determining how things turn out. If nutrition and hydration are withdrawn, we will never know whether the patient would have recovered some degree of brain function. If the patient had recovered some degree of brain function, the rightness of the decision to withdraw food and water could have been called into question. We are left with nothing but counter-factuals, and no escape from the paradox of moral luck.

Although I accept that none of Andrews's patients regained full higher consciousness, I want to use his study as a 'what-if?': something more than a hypothetical but less than clear proof that the diagnosis of persistent vegetative state is never appropriate. To put things the other way round, if there is any conceivable probability above 0.0 that consciousness may not have departed forever, then the argument from the permanent alienation of consciousness must fail. But exactly what does that failure entail?

First, then, let us consider the effect of Andrews's findings that persistent vegetative state does not necessarily mean the permanent extinction of all higher cerebral function. The probability that a PVS patient will ever regain full mental function remains infinitesimal, but that is not the same as zero, particularly when we consider the magnitude of the decision to terminate life support. In the parallel metaphor of eternal damnation, as Pascal argued, probabilities are irrelevant, dwarfed by the infinite magnitude of the possible loss. Any probability of such a loss is intolerable, if greater than zero. Pascal's strategic argument for belief in God hinges on the power of an infinite loss to cancel out even the slightest probability. If God does exist, and if he punishes those who do not believe in Him with eternal damnation, the loss entailed by non-belief is infinite. If we withhold belief and continue to sin, the minor rewards and pleasures of the non-believer's life will be cancelled out by the infinite loss of salvation. However slight the chance of God's existence may appear to the non-believer, even that infinitesimal probability is worth 'wagering' on, since the reward of a correct 'guess' will be eternal life. No matter how compelling the evidence against God's existence may appear, if there is the slightest shred of doubt in the mind of the atheist, she should recognize that belief is the better 'bet'. An infinitely great utility, positive or negative, cancels out the tiniest probability.

Once we admit that there is some possibility, however infinitesimal, of the patient in persistent vegetative state regaining some degree of conscious mental function, Pascal's Wager also applies. If death is regarded as an infinite loss, then we should be wary of allowing the patient to die if there is even the slimmest probability of recovery. If that is so, then the two arms of the paradox sketched in the introduction to this chapter are not really comparable. When a doctor withdraws treatment from a patient diagnosed as being in persistent vegetative state, that action inflicts an infinite loss, as against the more limited losses of remaining in that state for what may be many years. That is a heavier responsibility than maintaining the patient in persistent vegetative state through artificially supplied nutrition and hydration. We should therefore beware of following that path – particularly because, if all doctors do so for all patients diagnosed as being in persistent vegetative state, there will be no countervailing body of data which may provide us with better calibrated probabilities about whether patients really can recover some degree of consciousness, and with a firmer basis for the diagnosis of persistent vegetative state.

Like many medical ethicists, I initially supported the *Bland* decision, but I now find myself compelled to rethink my position. Here is where my rethinking stops short, however. I am uncertain as to whether death can properly be described as an infinite loss. On the one hand I want to say that it can, because clearly no other gain or pleasure can henceforth be experienced; all other pains and pleasure are in that sense finite, and death greater than any other loss. Yet, on the other hand, people do willingly risk their lives in calculations that seem to imply death is not infinite, but rather something we can set against probabilities in the usual expected-value sort of equation. And of course we also talk about 'fates worse than death', implying that death is not infinitely bad. Many people might regard continued existence in persistent vegetative state as just such a fate.

In the previous version of this book I considered the same problem in relation to nuclear deterrence, where I argued that 'what we face in the nuclear holocaust is the possibility of a loss so vast as to wipe out probability calculations.'[11] Even that may not strictly speaking be an infinite loss, however – not to a believer, certainly, for whom this world is finite, as are individual lives. I feel happier in making a slightly more bounded claim for both cases: that the possibility that the loss *may* be infinite should be enough to deter the prudent policy-maker or doctor. As I argued earlier, 'That will be the appropriate course for prudential reasoning: to know its own limits.'[12]

What do I mean by that in relation to withdrawal of treatment? The *Bland* case gave clinicians legal and practical cause to think that they could ignore the branch of the outcome luck conundrum in which the patient recovers. It would now be prudent, and ethical too, to stop ignoring that set of outcomes. If they occur, they are arguably worse than the other set, because the responsibility involved for the doctor who terminates life-sustaining treatment is heavier than that involved in continuing to treat.

Why this is so does not depend solely on 'evidence': in any case, if all doctors withdraw life-sustaining treatment, there will be no 'evidence' about recovery from persistent vegetative state. It is true for analytical reasons, because of the Pascal's Wager parallel, and also for legal ones: because failure to treat a patient for whom treatment is not certain to be futile and to whom one has a duty of care is criminally liable. I am not willing to say that doctors must always offer life-sustaining nutrition and hydration to patients in PVS because, just as such treatment cannot be known in advance to be certainly futile, likewise it cannot be known in advance to be certain to do good. But there is an imbalance between the two arms of that statement, and between the two sets of outcomes for which doctors may be held responsible. It is in fact that imbalance which allows us to escape from the moral luck paradox: doctors are not equally responsible, whichever branch they choose, if that choice turns out badly. They are more responsible for cutting short the life of someone in their care who might conceivably have made some degree of mental recovery than for continuing to maintain someone in a 'living death'. The British Medical Association guidelines on withdrawal and withholding of life-sustaining care treat PVS differently from other diagnoses, requiring a year before treatment can be withdrawn. This seems a good balance, reflecting the imbalance between the two arms of the statement and the two sorts of outcomes for which doctors are responsible.

To escape the chilling effect on agents' responsibility of moral luck, we should try to avoid the situation in which we will never know whether someone whose nutrition and hydration are taken away would have made some sort of recovery.[13] As has been said of irreversibility as the criterion of brain death, such a judgement 'requires the benefit of some significant degree of hindsight'.[14] It therefore raises the same paradoxes about justification by hindsight that we encountered early in chapter 1, concerning Williams's example of Gauguin. We do not generally think that agents can be held responsible for the sort of outcome ill-luck that can be known only in hindsight. Thus we risk undermining the central notion that doctors can ever be held accountable for withdrawal of life-sustaining treatment if we accept that PVS patients' chances of recovery could be known only in hindsight, but simultaneously allow doctors to discontinue nutrition and hydration for patients in PVS. To minimize the effect of the paradox of moral luck, we should try to minimize the number of situations in which hindsight is the only guide. It now looks, with the hindsight provided by Andrews's research, as if there might have been something more than a zero chance of Bland's recovering some degree of consciousness, or at least as if the clinicians should have acted with that possibility in mind.

Some might say that death would still have been in Bland's best interests, whether or not there was some minimal probability of his recovering a degree of consciousness. The Law Lords were in the main quite careful, however, *not* to state that death would be in Bland's best interests: once they had accepted that he had lost all features of human agency, they ruled that he could have no best interests.

> The distressing truth which must not be shirked is that the proposed conduct is not in the best interests of Anthony Bland, for he has no best interests of any kind.[15]

This necessary manoeuvre got the Lords round the paradox of appealing to Bland's best interests by ordering withdrawal of life-sustaining treatment. That would have been problematic, because the court would have been appealing to the best interests of someone who would no longer exist or have best interests, once the judgment was followed. Instead the court held that the entity that could have best interests had already ceased to exist before the judgment was made. So the argument that death would have been in Bland's best interests is internally contradictory.

Once recovery of some features of legal personality and human agency is again on the cards, it must then follow that the best interests of persons in persistent vegetative state do have to be considered. The implications are again that treatment of patients in PVS is to be preferred over non-treatment, as it is a general principle of English law – what one might call the 'fail-safe' principle – that medical treatment is normally presumed to be in the patient's best interests, even though the competent adult patient may refuse life-saving treatment.[16] This is why children of Jehovah's Witnesses will be given blood transfusions against their parents' will: the criterion is the patient's best interests. Normally parents are presumed to act in the best interests of a child, but when they refuse a life-saving transfusion, that presumption fails, and the court will order that the child should be transfused without parental consent.[17]

Given that Tony Bland, although an adult, was not competent to reject or accept treatment, his best interests, if defined as medical best interests, would presumably have dictated continuation of hydration and nutrition. The only way out of this bind would be to say that continued survival was not in his medical best interests, but if there is a possibility of recovery, however remote, it is hard to see how this position could be maintained. We could not escape from the dilemma by denying that someone who is dying – if we view Bland as dying – can still have best interests. Clearly they can: we do not look favourably on moving patients at death's door out of hospital, on the grounds that they represent a waste of resources. Indeed, in some cases we spend more on their care than on those who have good prospects of recovery, and this is right and proper in view of the dignity of dying people: hospice care is an expensive option, but in my opinion it is very much the right option.[18]

There are many other instances in death and dying of the role of risk, luck and certainty. In the much-debated conjoined twins case decided in September 2000,[19] the Court of Appeal was confronted with this question: is it right to hasten the death of someone who is certain to die in order to benefit someone else whose life can be saved by the death of the first person? The key variable in the Court of Appeal judgment seemed to be the certainty of the first twin's impending death – and of the second twin's being dragged down to death with her unless surgery could be performed to separate them. With surgery, the second twin was deemed to have a reasonable chance of life, although not absolute certainty of survival. Here the judgment of certainty seemed to be better founded than in the *Bland* case, or at least in the *Bland* case as we can now view it, with the additional knowledge afforded by Andrews's research. But in the *Bland* judgment the question was allowing to die, not killing. Even if the eventual death of the first twin was certain, does that certainty justify killing her in order to save her sister? The leading judge, Mr Justice Ward, argued that it did, on the principle of self-defence, but to many that argument was flawed by the fact that the baby was not actually defending herself. Even if those who came to her defence – the doctors – could be construed as acting in her aid, that duty conflicted with their duty of care to the first twin.

The role of chance in decisions about death and dying was also highlighted in the arguments made in favour of permitting assisted suicide in two companion Supreme Court decisions handed down in 1997.[20] In both cases the court reversed two earlier circuit court of appeal decisions declaring state statutes forbidding assisted suicide unconstitutional. One of the appeal judgments had been made on Fourteenth Amendment equal protection grounds: that it was discriminatory to deny the right to die to patients who were unable to kill themselves, when patients on life-support systems, such as Nancy Cruzan, have a constitutional right to have that support terminated. This sort of argument is often heard, in fact: in the December 2001 UK High Court case of Diane Pretty, a patient in the terminal stages of motor neurone disease, it was alleged to be unfair to deny Mrs Pretty the same rights to kill herself that an able-bodied person would have enjoyed, if that is the right word. The argument was rejected by the court.[21] The other US judgment also drew on the Fourteenth Amendment, but this time the due process clause: the argument here was that the state may not interfere with persons' liberty rights – including the right to die – without due process of the law. It is the equal protection argument which is more interesting from the viewpoint of risk and luck.

We may well feel that it is somehow unfair that some people contract motor neurone disease, or that they suffer paralysis in a car crash, or whatever other reason prevents them from undertaking suicide without assistance. That sense of injustice, about their loss of the ability to control their own fate, exists in addition to our feeling that having the condition is unfair in the first place. Apart from treating the condition, there is little that we can do about the second kind of unfairness, which results from an act of God or nature (assuming that the patient has not 'brought the condition on himself', which risks blaming the victim). The operations of chance and luck are highly visible here: luck in antecedent circumstances (whether or not one retains the physical power to control one's own death) and luck in the decisions that have to be faced (whether to seek someone else's help in dying). In the American context, of course, luck also plays a part in whether indigent dying patients have a right to adequate health care, including the services of the doctor who would presumably assist their suicide, and indeed Justice Breyer made exactly this point.[22]

But even if the situation of those who cannot kill themselves is somehow unfair, is it the job of doctors to put that inequity right? Daniel Callahan has drawn attention to a crucial distinction in his much-cited remark 'Your right to die doesn't imply my duty to kill.' In another distinction, introduced in chapter 1, I drew on Dworkin's comparison between option luck and brute luck. Option luck is a matter of deliberate choice in risk acceptance; brute luck involves the risks we do not choose. Developing motor neurone disease, or a similarly incapacitating condition that prevents the sufferer from taking her own life, is clearly a matter of brute luck. But in chapter 1 I argued that responsibility can attach only to outcome luck.[23] Doctors are not responsible, any more than patients are, for matters of brute luck, and therefore they are not responsible for putting matters of brute luck right. They may well feel regret that they cannot do more to aid the MND sufferer who cannot take her own life (although the acceptance of the doctrine of double effect in both US and UK common law means that they can actually do quite a lot to relieve pain and suffering, even if pain relief hastens the sufferer's demise).[24] But they should not feel remorse because they cannot rectify all the 'unfair' operations of fate.

Advance directives

Let us return again to the Bland case. In chapter 4, when I said that doctors should not subject patients to risks without consent, but are not responsible for ill-luck in outcomes if risks have been properly communicated, I also said that I would deal later with the question of what 'properly communicated' means. Although Andrews details some examples of minimal success in communicating with patients in persistent vegetative state, it seems abundantly clear that no one could communicate with Tony Bland, not even his dedicated consultant, Jim Howe, or his equally diligent family. The same problem arises with demented patients and many others who lack the mental capacity needed to give an informed consent or refusal. Are we then obliged to jettison the position I developed earlier, where incompetent patients are concerned? If so, then the power and range of my argument will be considerably weakened. It will be only in the case of competent patients who can give an informed consent, or refusal, that responsibility for ill-luck in outcomes can be transferred from doctor to patient.

One way around this difficulty would be advance directives or 'living wills'. By specifying in advance of losing competence which treatments one would want to refuse on becoming incompetent, we could retain the same structure for transferring responsibility. If Tony

Bland had executed an advance directive before his accident, he could have specified whether or not he would want artificial nutrition and hydration to be continued. Indeed, Lord Goff noted in his opinion that 'the same principle [that a competent patient's refusal must be respected] applies when the patient's refusal to give consent has been expressed at an earlier date, before he became unconscious or otherwise incapable of communicating it.'[25] The decision would still be his, and would still be binding once he lost the power of communication. All that happens in that case is that the transfer of responsibility for risks occurs at an earlier stage in the doctor–patient interaction.

In many ways I think this is an attractive solution, and I have argued elsewhere that even people with intermittent or chronic mental illness should be allowed to execute advance directives.[26] But there are still a number of problems. Despite a series of consultative documents from the Law Commission and the Lord Chancellor's Department,[27] there is at present no statutory basis for advance directives in English law, although case law has established the principle that a competent adult can refuse treatment in advance of becoming incompetent. That much has been made clear by the case of Mr C, a long-term patient in a secure hospital who refused amputation of a gangrenous foot, and who sought successfully to prevent the hospital from operating should he become comatose as a result of his illness.[28] It has not yet been established whether advance refusal would be binding once the patient had become incompetent, since that never actually occurred in Mr C's case, but the common law position is believed to be that advance refusal which is clearly established and applicable in the circumstances would indeed be binding.[29] In the United States advance directives were first established by statute in California in 1976, and were further encouraged by the Patient Self-Determination Act of 1991, which required any hospital receiving federal funding (including Medicare and Medicaid) to raise with incoming patients the possibility of executing an advance directive. Although in England living wills are limited to 'information directives', most US states also admit 'proxy directives', in which, rather than specifying particular treatments that are not to be administered, the decision about whether to withhold or withdraw treatment is left to the patient's nominated substitute decision-maker. Nevertheless, the percentage of people who actually execute a living will hovers around a mere 10 per cent, with slightly higher take-up in groups such as HIV-positive patients who have good reason to be aware of their mortality.[30] Young men such as Tony Bland, with no previous history of illness, are highly unlikely to number among the tiny minority who do take out an advance directive.

The most interesting problems, in terms of this book, centre not so much on such practicalities as on 1) risk and luck in outcomes and 2) luck in character. First, I shall look at risk. In his article 'Betting your life: an argument against certain advance directives', Christopher James Ryan examines why we should not be bound by the young person's high-flown scorn for prolonging life at all costs once we are actually seriously ill. Now one might think that if that really is the prevalent view among young people, the percentage taking out advance directives rejecting treatment would be very much higher than it actually is. Nevertheless Ryan offers an ingenious psychological argument which is well worth rehearsing here, bearing as it does on this book's themes of risk and luck. Ryan offers the following hypothetical scenario, concerning another sort of wager than Pascal's:

> A long time ago, in a country far far away, there lived a very wise old king. The king was a very ethical man and his subjects were very happy. Everyone lived together in perfect harmony and times were generally regarded as good.
>
> One day the king introduced a new law. The law allowed his subjects to enter into a mysterious wager. Those who won the wager would receive a rich reward, but those who lost would be put to death. Entry into the wager was entirely voluntary and despite the dire consequences of losing many took up the challenge. To win, a contestant had only correctly to answer an apparently straightforward question. The question was known to all participants before they entered and all who took up the challenge were sure that they knew the answer and could not lose. Strangely, even the king's ethicists had no objection to the introduction of the law and in fact praised the king for his wisdom and progressiveness. The ethicists also believed that the answer to the question was obvious and focused only on the rich reward.
>
> Unfortunately, however, many contestants got the answer wrong. They lost the wager and were put to an early and needless death. The question that caused so much difficulty was this: 'Even though you are now well and healthy, imagine yourself in a situation where you have a terminal illness and are temporarily confused or unconscious. Imagine that whilst you are in this state your doctors give you a choice; either they will treat you to the best of their ability and you may recover some of your health for some undefined period, or they will treat you conservatively and, though they will ensure that you are in no pain, they will not attempt to save your life. If you were in this situation, what would you want to doctors to do?'[31]

Now there are a number of flaws in this intriguing parallel. Failing to treat is not the same as killing; if it were, doctors would be criminally liable whenever they fail to do everything that could conceivably be done. Furthermore, avoiding a prolonged death cannot really be compared with a 'rich reward': at best, it is the absence of a loss. It may well be true, however, that even ethicists have focused too much on avoiding a prolonged and undignified death, just as the king's ethicists are obsessed with the 'rich reward'. Daniel Callahan has argued that American bioethics in particular has been too ready to accept advance directives as the 'magic bullet' to cure the ills of overtreatment and overuse of technology that continue to bedevil the American health care system, with its financial incentives for treating at all costs.[32]

Where Ryan's metaphor works best is in its elucidation of how little we know about our own preferences. Although 'informed' consent is rarely understood as being informed about one's own values, rather than about treatment information, Ryan focuses on how poorly we perform when asked to put ourselves into our own shoes many years down the line, when we are terminally ill. But this is exactly what advance directives require us to do. Whether this sort of failure really is irrational is also a major concern in the work of Derek Parfit: in particular, the discussion in *Reasons and Persons* of whether it is irrational to give no weight to one's past desires.[33]

Like the citizens of the mythical kingdom, many people answer 'wrongly', Ryan claims, when asking themselves about their future treatment and non-treatment preferences. In particular, we are likely radically to underestimate our desire for continued treatment once we become ill, especially in the final stages of a terminal illness. In Ryan's view this failure is due to denial, but it does not really matter what the psychological basis for it might be, to the extent that it is supported by evidence. One study, for example, found that cancer patients with potentially curative treatment expressed a stronger desire for euthanasia than those whose prognosis was actually poorer.[34] Similarly, another study, examining the stability of future treatment preferences, found that those who had been hospitalized, had an accident or lost their mobility expressed stronger preferences for further treatment than before their illness.[35] Completed suicide attempts are also more common at the time when a terminal diagnosis is first imparted than later in illness, when pain and suffering are actually worse[36] (although of course patients may also lose the physical capacity to commit suicide as the disease progresses). Although he does not offer a systematic survey of evidence and counter-evidence,[37] Ryan argues that all these studies point towards the same conclusion: that we are wrong about what must be construed to be our 'true wishes' about treatment and non-treatment when we are actually terminally ill. We will probably want treatment to continue, once it is sooner rather than later that we face the stark choice between further treatment and death.

If we really are as poor as Ryan claims at predicting how our own preferences are likely to change once we are diagnosed as terminally ill, then there might be grounds for caution in hoping that advance directives can perform the same transfer of responsibility for ill-luck in outcomes as a contemporaneous consent does in my model. The conclusion Ryan draws is that certain advance directives should in fact be prohibited, namely those rejecting treatment in advance, in a situation where the patient is temporarily incompetent but that incapacity is potentially reversible. I have already said that I do not consider this parallel with the 'being executed' arm of the wager really works. Nor am I persuaded that the only sorts of treatment decisions that may be said to suffer from insufficient self-knowledge, and more broadly from insufficient understanding of treatment information, are advance ones. In chapter 4 I mentioned the study of twenty cardiac patients interviewed before and after their operation, of whom precious few could remember having been told and having understood utterly crucial information for giving an informed consent. But we do not make the right to give an informed consent contingent on adult patients' understanding of risks: rather, we uphold a general presumption of competence in adults, no matter how badly they understand their own preferences or the information doctors give them.[38] So although Ryan's statistics are cautionary, and the wager metaphor compelling, I think his policy argument ultimately fails, leaving the possibility of advance directives as a valid means of transferring responsibility for ill-luck in outcomes from doctor to patient.

Ryan's argument also points in another direction, however: this time towards luck in character. In the final part of this section, I want to consider questions about identity and advance preferences in greater detail. Let us begin by revisiting Gauguin's dilemma, and my discussion of it in chapter 1. There I drew attention to this problem:

> The Gauguin who must assess his own talent as an artist, back in Paris, is one who has not yet sounded the full range of his artistic talents; he is in an important sense a different person from the Gauguin he might

become if he goes to Tahiti. Since his knowledge is imperfect, and since he can know only in hindsight, as the Tahiti Gauguin, whether his decision as the Paris Gauguin was justified, the problem of moral luck in the decision he must make in Paris is serious and inescapable.

What may have seemed a rather esoteric argument to the reader of chapter 1 is brought home with immediate clinical force by advance directives. By the time my advance directive takes effect, on my losing the capacity to accept or reject treatment, I may in a sense be a different person. That eventuality may occur in a dramatic way – if I become severely demented – or simply because I change my mind progressively over time as my illness progresses, perhaps for the reasons Ryan suggests. If I really am a different person at the time my advance directive takes effect from the person I am when I draw it up, then effectively my earlier self is directing the treatment decisions of my later self. English law does not allow another adult – even close kin, which I suppose I may call myself in my relation to my later self – to direct the treatment decisions of any adult, competent or not. Law in the United States is more flexible about proxy decision-makers but, whatever the legal position, the ethical problem remains. The fear that people taking out advance directives may change their minds, but fail to record that change in the directive, has been cited as a cautionary note against living wills by many commentators,[39] but the problem is worsened if we actually conceive of the later self as a different person from the earlier self.[40] To hearken back to the language of the Gauguin example, since my knowledge is imperfect, and since I can know only in hindsight, as the dying me, whether my decision as the healthy me was justified, the problem of moral luck in the decision I must make as the healthy me is serious and inescapable.

This can also be construed as a matter of luck in character. I cannot know in advance whether and how my character will change once I lose mental capacity. Although I like to believe myself to be the same, unified personality now as I will be then, dementia and other forms of incapacity may vastly alter my character in ways that I cannot predict. That change may not be odious to me once I lose capacity, but the prospect of it is upsetting to me now, not least because of my Kantian sympathies. Dementia is a particularly poignant aspect of the problem identified by Margaret Walker in chapter 1: that the Kantian attempt to 'drive responsibility inside' to acts of the will or character, as a way to evade moral luck, is threatened by the way in which chance events can also determine the inner life.[41]

Yet perhaps this is to exaggerate. Our law and social life are founded on the principle that we respect a person's past preferences, and indeed that a person can be bound by her past preferences: this is what promises and contract are all about.[42] We do not worry unduly about whether she is a different person now from then, provided she was an adult when she made the promise or signed the contract (presumably because we do think that people's identities alter more between childhood and maturity, although, as I have noted elsewhere, stable preferences and characters may be formed well before the legal age of majority).[43] If we have reason to believe that the contract or promise is invalid because it was signed under duress, or was not fully voluntary, we may exempt her from it, but without speculating that she is actually a different person now from her past self. Again, we may allow that she was less than perfectly informed at the time she made the contract, and perhaps exempt her from its performance for that reason, particularly if she was deliberately deceived – but we need not view her as a different person then from the person she is now. So why should we treat promises such as advance directives made now, and binding in the future, any differently? We need not view the future person as a different person, with an entirely different character, in order to allow her the right to change her mind, even if her mind is a mere shadow of its former self.

In an earlier article (co-written with Julian Savulescu) I used the example of Ulysses and the Sirens, a classic example of an advance directive. With his crew, Ulysses (Odysseus) was about to pass the Island of the Sirens,

> whose beautiful voices enchanted all who sailed near. [They]...had girls' faces but birds' feet and feathers... and sat and sang in a meadow among the heaped bones of sailors they had drawn to their death.[44]

Wishing to hear the fabled song but also to survive, Ulysses instructed his men to bind him to the mast, to plug their own ears with beeswax, and to lash him more tightly still to the mast if he demanded to be released as they passed the Island of the Sirens. This tactic worked, like most of wily Ulysses's stratagems. In our analysis, Savulescu and I identified three relevant desires in the case of Ulysses:

D1 Ulysses desires to live.
D2 Ulysses desires to hear the song from afar.
D3 Ulysses desires to hear the song very closely.

At the time he instructed his men to bind him to the mast and to stop up their own ears, Ulysses possessed desires D1 and D2. At the time of passing the island, he changed from D2 to D3. Does that necessarily entail the disappearance of D1? – and of the Ulysses who formed the original desire? No, we argued: D1 persisted, but was dominated by D3. To claim that D1 had disappeared would imply that our lives are nothing but a succession of momentary desires; but the mere fact that Ulysses could form the project of preserving his life while experiencing the Sirens' song shows that contradictory desires may co-exist, and can be reconciled by means of a long-term strategy.[45]

The capacity to form such a strategy, and to entertain conflicting desires, is typical of human agency. Although the maddened Ulysses who screams to be released from his bonds is different from the cunning Ulysses who foresees his own mental incapacity, it is the ability to foresee how he may change, and to take action accordingly, that actually confirms Ulysses' agency. The same is true of the person who foresees dementia or other forms of mental incapacity and makes provision accordingly, through an advance directive. Rather than undermining attributions of responsibility, in a manner that is hopelessly undermined by moral luck, one might equally well argue that advance directives demonstrate a particularly responsible form of agency, and that they indicate continuity of agency rather than a series of separate selves. So we can avoid problems about luck in successive characters that way, and also the Gauguin-style problems identified by Williams.

What might make us uncomfortable about the Ulysses parallel, however, is the practical implication that the incompetent person must be held to her advance directive, particularly to withdrawal of life support, even if she still appears to be enjoying life. Savulescu and I wrote: 'It is not merely because Ulysses did desire to live, or because he will desire to live, but because he now desires to live that we restrain him.'[46] The Ulysses parallel breaks down at this point. I cannot say: 'It is not merely because the incompetent patient did desire to die, or because she will desire to die, but because she now desires to die that we constrain her to do so.' Indeed, I want to argue that we should not constrain a mentally incapacitated person to die if she experiences pleasure in her life as she lives it now, if, so far as clinicians can tell, she desires to live on. So we need to examine briefly, in concluding this section, what it is in the now-incapacitated person's present preferences that ought to be respected.

The answer seems to be the very fact that they are present preferences. Savulescu and I argued that it is especially important to respect present preferences in a liberal democratic society; that preferences should be construed as predispositions; and that a person who is now incompetent may still have relevant predispositions that should be respected.[47] On the dispositional analysis we offered, an advance directive should be respected only if it represents an enduring present preference. Of course there will be many cases where it is impossible to ascertain the patient's present preference, and where there is no evidence to indicate that the present preference differs from the past preference, the past preference should be respected. Where there is no evidence of either past or present preferences in favour of treatment withdrawal, then, on the account developed earlier, in which not treating leads to weightier problems of moral luck than treating, clinicians should err in favour of treatment, particularly with an uncertain diagnosis such as PVS.

As I wrote at the beginning of the chapter, 'when a doctor withdraws treatment from a patient diagnosed as being in persistent vegetative state, that action inflicts an infinite loss, as against the more limited losses of remaining in that state for what may be many years. That is a heavier responsibility than maintaining the patient in persistent vegetative state through artificially supplied nutrition and hydration. We should therefore beware of following that path.'

6

Moral Luck and the Allocation of Health Care Resources

Does moral luck apply to the allocation of dialysis machines? To the provision of scarce beds in an intensive care unit for children with heart conditions? To organ transplants? To distributing the scarce resource of nurse time? I want to show that it does, but, conversely, I think we can also apply findings from resource allocation back to the general paradox of moral luck. As elsewhere in the six practical chapters of the book, there is a two-way relationship between practical and theoretical ethics.

Although questions about resource allocation are generally treated under the rubric of distributive justice, the first part of this chapter, on the 'micro' level, will concentrate instead on individual agency, responsibility and identity. This approach corresponds to the individual practitioner's needs in making 'micro' decisions, for example in the allocation of nurse time. The concepts of regret and remorse will be considered: what happens when an allocation decision goes wrong? I argue in favour of a randomized system of resource allocation as the only means of avoiding overwhelming regret and remorse if ill-luck in outcomes occurs, or if some patients are disadvantaged because of luck in antecedent circumstances.

In the second part of the chapter I turn to public policy, at the 'macro' level, and defend my randomized model of resource allocation against the trend towards evidence-based medicine (EBM). Whereas EBM seeks to maximize information, random allocation, rather like Rawls's Veil of Ignorance, deliberately suppresses some information that might be thought relevant to resource allocation decisions. Does this make the randomized model an ineffective decision-making model in the wider context? I also look at social rather than medical criteria for rationing at the level of public policy.

In passing I shall also be considering some issues at the 'macro-macro' level of *global* resource allocation.

The 'micro' level

One way of conceptualizing what is going on in 'tragic choices'[1] about allocation of a scarce resource between parties, each of whom has a reasonable claim to it, is whether the agent's responsibility is

- to get the optimal distribution 'right' in light of available resources
- to make the allocation decision in the 'right' manner.

These two contrasting approaches can be mapped against consequentialism, virtue ethics and Kantianism. The first approach, focusing on outcomes, is consequentialist; the second could be either Kantian, if the 'right' manner is that which maximizes patient autonomy and demonstrates respect for persons, or compatible with virtue ethics, if the 'right' manner is that which would be demonstrated by a virtuous practitioner. From the argument in chapters 2 and 3, the reader will deduce that I do not favour the first approach, and that will turn out to be because I think it leaves the practitioner vulnerable to ill-luck in outcomes. That was my strategy in the two previous chapters: where informed consent is concerned, I argued, the practitioner can avoid the depredations of ill-luck in *outcomes* by concentrating on the *process* of obtaining informed consent, so that a meaningful consent transfers responsibility for ill-luck in outcomes from doctor to patient. The structure of the argument was set out in chapter 4; chapter 5 tested it against some hard cases – for example, in relation to dying patients who can no longer give an informed consent.

What about making resource allocation decisions? To put the argument in terms of Nagel's maxim, is it possible for the practitioner to act in a way that would not have to be revised in the light of outcomes? What will it mean for the person allocating scarce resources on the 'micro' level, in the context of everyday clinical decisions, to act in an outcome-impervious way? Does it have something to do with getting it right *this* time? That would be in line with the practitioner's duty of care towards each individual patient. And it would also be consistent with the impetus in Nesson's example of the 25 prisoners, where it was not good enough to employ any means to get an overall figure of 24 convictions and one acquittal. Each man was being tried on his own, and, if we wanted to respect basic legal principles, each deserved to have his case kept separate from any considerations about the aggregate. We had to get each trial right; in each prisoner's case, we had to get it right this time.

What made it wrong to breach the ethical/legal principle of prior innocence was not that this was a life-and-death decision. It would still have been wrong in a jurisdiction that lacked the death penalty. Similarly, in health resource allocation, the importance of 'getting it right' will be as great in less dramatic instances, such as the allocation of nursing time on non-acute wards, as in the life-and-death cases such as heart transplants.

The criterion in the Nesson example was not getting the mathematical conundrum right in each case, or even for the aggregate, but rather maintaining the principle of prior innocence. We were unable to 'get it right' in mathematical terms: the only solution appeared to be acquitting all 25 prisoners, even though we knew that 24 were guilty. So 'getting it right' *this* time may mean respecting personal autonomy or some other ethical criterion that occupies a similar position to the principle of innocent until proven guilty in law. Or it may mean acting compassionately, impartially, or according to whatever virtue is appropriate to resource-allocation decisions. Because virtue ethics concerns what sort of person it is right to be, rather than what it is right to do, it, too, will suggest that getting it right *this* time is possible only in terms of the wider context of what sort of person it is good to be in *all* one's professional decisions. Either way, the focus widens from this particular outcome, and that itself mitigates the effect of ill-luck in how the immediate case turns out.

But, as in the Nesson example, there remains a tension between individual and group, even though we are concerned in this part of the chapter primarily with the individual case. The clinician owes a duty of care to the individual patient. What is the appropriate reaction for the practitioner who 'gets it wrong' in this particular case? We shall need to revisit the discussion of regret and remorse in chapter 3, asking whether clinicians should feel regret, remorse, neither or both when a scarce health-care resource must be denied to patients in their care. In particular, how should the doctor feel about the case in which the outcome turns out badly – the patient who did not get the kidney that was 'wasted' on someone who died shortly thereafter, the relatives of the patient who did get the kidney but who died after 'false hopes' had been raised?

It may help to make clinicians' duties less all-encompassing if we make a distinction between deciding how much of a scarce health-care resource will be produced and deciding how it will be allocated.[2] Here Dworkin's distinction between brute and option luck is relevant. We might well want to claim that brute luck decides how many kidneys will be available, and how prevalent kidney failure will be. Agents' responsibilities are second-order, in that case. Clinicians do not set the probability machine rolling, and, to the extent that it rolls of its own accord, 'deciding how much of a scarce health-care resource will be produced' misrepresents the kidney case.

Against that reasoning, deciding how much of a health 'good' will be produced can certainly be a matter of deliberate choice, and hence of outcome luck, in instances other than the kidney example. Deciding how many nurse hours will be available, for example, is a policy choice, not just a demographic fact dictated by the number of eighteen-year-old women with the appropriate qualifications and desire to enter nurse training. In the late 1980s the UK government implicitly recognized this truth by mounting a large-scale advertising campaign to convince more women to enter nursing, in order to counter the demographic decline in this cohort. (Choosing to spend resources on advertising rather than increased salaries or resources was also a policy decision, of course.)

At the clinical rather than the governmental level, there will always remain resource allocation decisions that cannot be set down to mere brute luck, and that really do appear to be cases where outcome luck is relevant. How can practitioners decide such cases without becoming mired in remorse if the choice turns out badly? Elsewhere[3] I have offered a fivefold typology:

1   *Clinical criteria: prognosis*, the resource should go to those with the best chance of recovery (utilizing the input with maximum productive efficiency). This basis for decision-making has the apparent advantage of bypassing subjective considerations. It interprets the Aristotelian dictum of treating equals equally as treating alike those who are equal with respect to observable evidence-based criteria. Evidence-based medicine and the QALY (quality-adjusted life year) approach that underpins the deliberations of the UK's National Institute for Clinical Excellence are guided by this approach (although an element of subjectivity is also built into QALYs insofar as they record patient preferences for one state of health above another).

2   *Clinical criteria: diagnosis*, the resource should go to those whose clinical need is most acute, even if their chances of recovery are not great. The most 'saveable' patient in terms of prognosis is unlikely to be the neediest or most severely ill patient in terms of diagnosis. Although 'objective' evidence is again used here, deliberate preference is given to patients whose treatment is not allocatively 'efficient'. Examples include palliative care and the aggressive treatment of very sick children (e.g. the Child B case).[4]

3   *Social criteria: past merit*, or 'social worth': here the choice is conceptualized in terms of the patient's past contribution to society, rather than clinical criteria. The possibility for this choice going 'wrong' is magnified by the subjectivity and sheer prejudice shown in the deliberations of the most egregious example of judging by past merit, the Seattle 'God' Committee. Formed in the early 1960s to produce guidelines for allocating what was then the scarce resource of haemodialysis, the committee took into account income, net worth, church membership and scout leadership. It was remarked that 'the Pacific Northwest is no place for a Henry David Thoreau with bad kidneys.'[5] To their credit, the members of the committee eventually recognized that they were producing biased judgements and disbanded the group.

4   *Social criteria: future merit*, or 'potential contribution': again, the choice is made not on 'objective' clinical criteria, but on the social criterion of some potential contribution to society, such as number of future work years. On this criterion, we should always prefer the young to the old, or at least the able-bodied young. Discrimination against the elderly or the disabled may result from applying this criterion. Another example of conflict between these two sets of social criteria is the decision during the North African campaign in World War II to give limited penicillin supplies to venereal disease sufferers, rather than to men wounded in battle. Honourably wounded soldiers might be seen as having greater past merit, but VD sufferers could recover more quickly if given the penicillin, and thus their potential contribution to the war effort was greater.

5   *Equality*: everyone should be treated equally in deciding how to share out the resource, regardless of need or merit. This criterion leads to a policy of randomizing allocation, or, more typically in the ordinary clinical context, to allocating resources on a first-come, first-served basis.

What moral luck problems are raised by medical criteria? Luck in antecedent circumstances is exemplified by the tricky way in which seemingly objective clinical criteria shade off into discrimination against the socially unfortunate. In the case of Derek Spence, at the Churchill Hospital in Oxford, the dialysis of a vagrant kidney patient was terminated because he was judged to be unable to follow the required diet if he was living on the streets. The consultant making the allocation decision claimed that he was acting purely on the patient's prognosis, but nurses challenged that claim, and the team decided to reinstate Spence in the dialysis programme. Another case, this time from the United States, concerned 'Baby Jesse', who needed a heart transplant. On medical grounds, he met the preliminary criteria, but his parents – unmarried teenagers with a criminal history and substance abuse problems – were judged unlikely to provide the necessary follow-up, such as punctual administration of immunosuppressive drugs. The clinicians who rejected Baby Jesse as a transplant candidate were accused of discriminating on social grounds, although they too maintained that they were merely allocating the extremely scarce resource of infant hearts according to objective medical criteria.

As Robert Veatch puts it:

> Parents with low intelligence or lack of a permanent residence or employment could probably be predicted statistically to provide a less supportive environment for a transplant patient. Studies could be done that would show that probability of successful transplant correlates with the recipient's socioeconomic status. Thus any of these apparently social criteria could be turned into medical criteria if they predicted the chance of a successful graft. The neat line between social and medical benefit collapses. Any allocation system that incorporates medical benefit could, in fact, be bootlegging social criteria.[6]

Comparing Italian and British methods of kidney and dialysis allocation, Guido Calabresi and Philip Bobbitt found that Italian doctors thought it a kind of 'bad faith' to claim that a purely clinical approach can avoid the operations of moral luck. British clinicians, they observed, believed that medical prognosis-derived criteria could evade ethical questions: 'The criteria are applied unswervingly, and damn the implications for general equality.'[7] By contrast, as described by Calabresi and Bobbitt,[8] the Italian system openly confronts the need to take an ethical stance in dealing with scarce medical resources. The moral creed that it seeks to reflect is absolute egalitarianism, meaning that favourable prognosis is abandoned as a criterion. This way of thinking leads to what many might regard as a result that allows the vagaries of chance full play. Under the Italian first-come, first-served system, a ninety-year-old patient with terminal renal cancer gets the kidney if she comes before the thirty-year-old with no other clinical symptoms than kidney failure. Surely this counts as failure and occasions regret, or even remorse?

Not if clinical appropriateness, particularly in terms of a more favourable prognosis, is itself regarded as conferred by chance – by luck in antecedent circumstances. Patients do not choose to suffer from terminal illness. As Calabresi and Bobbitt argue, 'Why should their shorter lives be measured against lives that would have been longer from no merit of their own?'[9] Although the language of merit is more normally used for social criteria, Calabresi and Bobbitt force us to recognize that having the 'right' prognosis, or indeed 'diagnosis', is itself a kind of unearned merit, conferred solely by the operations of chance. The reasoning parallels Rawls's treatment of intelligence, normally seen as an earned merit and therefore a legitimate basis for social preferment in job allocation, as instead being merely the gift of the Fates.[10] Similarly, the Italian model, as Calabresi and Bobbitt depict it, confronts luck head-on, drawing its fire by incorporating it – by *explicitly incorporating chance into the allocation mechanism*, in the form of randomized allocation or the principle of first come, first served.

If luck in antecedent circumstances matters, and if clinical suitability is a form of luck in antecedent circumstances, then it will be a form of outcome ill-luck when patients whose 'lives would have been longer from no merit of their own' are given preference over patients with a worse prognosis. This is the link between the two forms of moral luck that operate in resource allocation. That Italian doctors did take the possibility of this form of failure into account was clear from the interviews conducted by Calabresi with two directors of dialysis centres in Pisa and Florence.[11] These clinicians reiterated their loyalty to the 'principle of humane non-interference', or allocating resources among patients equally regardless of prognosis, even if as a result lives were lost 'unnecessarily'. There was regret in such cases, and a certain amount of hedging: the doctors normally reserved one or two emergency dialysis machines for the hard cases. And although equality on both social and medical grounds was the principle at these individual dialysis centres, it did not guide allocation at the level of public policy, where inequality predominated: there were many more dialysis places in the industrialized north than in the poorer south.[12] Still, such ill-chance is external to the clinicians' own 'project' (as Williams might put it) of treating all those who come to them on a basis of strict equality. It does not constitute personal failure for individual doctors, whose duty of care is to individual patients rather than a responsibility for the system as a whole. The failure to achieve countrywide fairness should not occasion remorse in the individual clinician.

Where there is conflict of life with life, lotteries have been held fairer than social criteria. In the shipwreck case of *US* v. *Holmes* (1841) the presiding judge ruled that a surviving crew member, Holmes, should not have collaborated with his shipmates in devising and implementing social criteria for deciding who among the survivors should be thrown off the lifeboat in order to lighten its load. Despite the likelihood that everyone would have died if someone had not been jettisoned, the judge refused to accept that the interests of individuals could be outweighed by more favourable consequences for the majority. In convicting Holmes of unlawful homicide, he also dismissed defence counsel's contention that the crew's method of selection – 'not to part man and wife, and not to throw over any woman' – was more ethical than a lottery. Only casting lots would have been a remedy that the law could sanction: 'in no other way than this or some like way are those having equal rights put on an equal footing, and in no other way is it possible to guard against partiality and oppression, violence and conflict.'[13] The law can be seen to be taking a deontological stance here, as so often:[14] there is a prior duty to ensure that everyone in equal need has an equal chance of the ultimate scarce resource, life.

Holmes is a particularly poignant case, deeply permeated by ill-luck in outcomes. The crew failed in their goal of preventing female deaths: two sisters jumped overboard to die with their brother, who was among the fourteen men pushed into the sea. Now of course the outcome of drawing straws, or some other lottery-like method, could also have been threatened by ill-luck: the brother might have drawn a short straw, the sisters long ones, and the outcome turned out the same. But would this have been cause for remorse in the lottery's organizers? Somehow this twist is less tragic: it undermines only the randomness of a lottery, not the moral value of preventing women's deaths. Of course any 'extra' death is tragic, but so are all the deaths and the entire situation. There is no good outcome, once we move beyond an extreme consequentialism in which any outcome whereby some are saved would be acceptable, no matter how it is decided who should die.

Some outcomes are worse than others not only for the dead, but also for the survivors. The ill-luck of the sisters choosing to die against the lottery's impersonal 'will' is less damaging to the organizers' moral 'project' than the sisters' death would have been to Holmes and his fellows, because the crew presumably held the sanctity of female life dear in a deep way that no one could feel about the randomness of lotteries' outcomes. The unlucky outcome of a lottery might have entailed regret; in legal terms – and, I argue, also in ethical ones – the crewmen's failure in *Holmes* was an occasion for remorse and the grounds for a criminal prosecution.

To clinicians the *Holmes* case – a nineteenth-century American decision about a shipwreck – may seem a very long way from everyday practice. A very typical case concerning a nurse allocating the resource of her scarce time serves to show that, on the contrary, randomization is a relevant and helpful concept, in conjunction with medical need (criterion 2) but not medical prognosis (criterion 1). The discussion so far should have made it plain why resource allocation by prognosis risks discrimination against patients whose antecedent circumstances are unlucky.

Robert Veatch and Sara Fry have developed a fictional example of a nurse who is confronted with the entirely typical case in which her duty is not to *the* patient, as the traditional codes have it, but rather to *patients* in the plural.[15] On a medical-surgical nursing-care unit, night nurse Clora Bingham has four needy patients. Mrs Robertson is a semi-comatose 83-year-old woman in need of suctioning every fifteen to twenty minutes to prevent a mucous plug from blocking her bronchi and causing respiratory failure. Mr Jablowski, 47, was admitted for observation after having presented with bloody bowel movements. Mr Hanson, 52, is a newly diagnosed diabetic on intravenous insulin, with unstable blood sugar levels, who needs frequent vital sign checks. The fourth patient, 35-year-old Mr Manfra, has no immediate medical needs but has been suicidal in the past. Fears that he might now repeat his suicidal behaviour have been heightened: he learned today that he has inoperable cancer of the spine.

What would randomization suggest? It seems unlikely that Clora Bingham can actually give all four patients equal amounts of her time, or that, even if she could, that kind of equality would be fair to all concerned. If she has to suction Mrs Robertson every fifteen minutes, she will be unable to give Mr Manfra the length of time he needs to talk. She will do him no good at all if she rushes off in the middle, and perhaps even some harm: he may become all the more depressed and angry at feeling abandoned. It looks very much as if her time is effectively indivisible, just like a kidney – even though a first reaction to the issue of nurse time as a scarce resource would be to say that it *is* divisible, unlike a kidney.

On criterion 1 (medical: prognosis) or 4 (social: future merit) Mrs Robertson seems the least important to help: her long-term prognosis is poor, and indeed she is already comatose. As is often the situation for hard-pressed health-care staff, Clora Bingham knows nothing about the patients' 'past' merit (criterion 3), and it would arguably breach professional guidelines for her to decide on that basis. On criterion 2 (medical: diagnosis) Mrs Robertson 'scores' highly, but so do Mr Hanson and Mr Manfra. Assuming that Mrs Robertson has not signed an advance directive rejecting this particular form of treatment (see chapter 5), it would be wrong to omit the procedure that is necessary for keeping her alive, even though she is almost certainly dying. However, whereas Mrs Robertson is almost certain to die if her needs are ignored, the same is not true of Mr Manfra. (Mr Hanson falls somewhere in between.) And if Mr Manfra does commit suicide, in a sense that will be his 'project' rather than hers.

On the other hand, an initial suicidal reaction to the diagnosis of inoperable cancer is sometimes followed by determination to live the remaining life to the full.[16] Could Clora Bingham be sure that Mr Manfra might not have changed his mind if he had had a bit of her time? Clearly not, but her choice of whether to give her limited time to him or to Mrs Robertson cannot be justified retrospectively by the outcome in either case. This is the argument from moral luck. Although her choice cannot be *justified* retrospectively, Nagel's maxim suggests that she will want to make a choice that she would not want to have *altered* even once the consequences were known.[17]

If Mr Manfra commits suicide, Clora Bingham will doubtless feel grief and regret, but there is no need for her to experience remorse, which would have to do with her failure as a moral agent. Mr Manfra's suicide is nothing to do with *her* failure; it is ultimately *his* decision as a moral agent. Her project of keeping all her patients alive and well, within the limitations of what medicine and nursing can do, would suffer as a result of Mr Manfra's suicide, but that entails only regret, not remorse. Mr Manfra can decide his own fate, assuming he retains mental capacity, as he seems to; the decision to commit suicide does not itself indicate lack of mental capacity, if there is no underlying mental pathology.[18]

In chapter 3 I introduced a third concept, Williams's notion of 'agent-regret', which has to do not with unfortunate external events but with the agent's own past actions that have gone wrong. Agent-regret recognizes that the success or failure of the agent's project is to some extent beyond the agent's control, but that the actions that set the project in train are her own. But in the case of Mr Manfra, the outcome is contingent mainly on his own actions as a moral agent, that is, his choice about whether to commit suicide. So, as I argued in chapter 3, agent-regret does not seem particularly useful in that sense.

However, I want to qualify the argument I made earlier, when I said that the notion of agent-regret is not helpful because it fails to take into account the duty of care that the health professional owes the individual patient, a duty to do one's utmost to get it right *this* time and not just in the long run. In cases of patients rather than patient, plural rather than singular – such as those typical of nurse time as a scarce resource – the concept of agent-regret may indeed be useful. Once we factor in Mrs Robertson's greater need, perhaps it might tell us something about how Clora Bingham would feel about the three remaining patients. Is it possible for Clora Bingham to act in such a way towards the three remaining patients that she would not later wish to have modified her decision in light of the outcome for each patient? She needs to be able to do so: nurses have been found to be able to cope with a patient's death most easily when they can tell themselves, with justice, that nothing more could have been done.[19]

I think the best way for Clora Bingham to achieve this goal is dividing her remaining time equally between the three men, on the principle of randomization. Clearly if any of the three men die, Clora Bingham will feel grief and regret, but she will not necessarily wish she had made the decision in a different way. If the checks and observations for Mr Jablowski and Mr Hanson allow substantial intervals, she may well be able to give Mr Manfra a longish period of time for a talk. There is no reason why she has to randomize her time mechanically: the principle does not require precisely five minutes per patient every fifteen minutes.

Dividing her time equally overall will be Clora Bingham's way of 'getting it right', whatever the outcome, for the three remaining patients. It will also be the procedure that spares her lengthy deliberations of each individual's precise claims to portions of her time – making that scarce resource even scarcer. Whatever the eventual outcome, the action she took in dividing her remaining time equally among the three remaining patients seems the right one. Conversely, if she had decided to give all her remaining time to the dramatic, sympathy-provoking case of Mr Manfra at the expense of Mr Jablowski's and Mr Hanson's somewhat more routine conditions, she would have had cause for agent-regret whatever the outcome, even if Mr Hanson had somehow escaped falling into a diabetic coma.

It has been said in defence of randomization that 'the more nearly total is the estimate to be made of an individual, and the more nearly the consequence determines life and death, the more unfit the judgement becomes for human reckoning.'[20] In the next section I want to argue that this is true at a societal level as well as for the individual clinician.

Knowing our limits: the 'macro' level

In this section I want to examine the notion of 'random justice' on the societal level.[21] Just as the concepts of 'moral' and 'luck' seemed to be antithetical, so might those of 'random' and 'justice' appear at first to be. Randomly redistributing wealth, for example, might mean that those who are already wealthy receive more, while the poor get nothing. How can this be just? It may be argued that, on the public policy level, decision-makers would be irresponsible in not making use of all available information in redistributing income and wealth.

A similar argument lies behind the development of evidence-based medicine (EBM), in which meta-analyses of randomized clinical trials are prepared systematically and may be used to guide health resource allocation. It is generally taken for granted that EBM will improve the quality of health care and make allocation of scarce resources more equitable, ending 'postcode prescribing' in which the patient's chances of obtaining a particular drug or treatment depend on the luck of where she lives. The UK's National Institute for Clinical Excellence (NICE) is charged with the brief of recommending whether or not certain treatments should be funded nationally by the NHS, taking into account impact on quality of life, relief of pain or disability, response rate, length of time between treatment and recurrence of disease, overall length of survival, and cost to the NHS over and above currently recommended treatments. The guidance issued by NICE is premised on the foundational notion in EBM, that if doctors prescribe the most effective treatments, based on meta-analyses of carefully conducted randomized clinical trials, patients will obviously benefit.[22]

One tension here, however, is between the doctor's duty of care to the *individual patient* and the *population focus* of EBM.[23] Neither of these is absolute, of course. A doctor's duty to an individual patient does not extend so far as to compromise the quality of care for other patients; she is not obliged to spend the last penny of the practice budget in order to maintain a child who is terminally ill with cancer, for example, if other patients will suffer. Conversely, although EBM deals in populations and probabilities, and although probabilities other than 1.00 and 0.00 do not tell us with absolute certainty what the prognosis is for this particular patient on this particular treatment, EBM may offer a finer-honed probability that will enable this particular patient to make a better-calibrated decision. Countries such as Norway, Sweden and Finland, with a long tradition of both socialized medicine and health technology assessment, certainly seem to see few tensions between providing the best available care to their entire population and EBM. It may be that, as the use of EBM becomes more sophisticated, there will also come to be less emphasis on uniform EBM-derived criteria for the entire patient population, so that the individual–population tension will diminish.[24] None the less, the legal and ethical emphasis is on the doctor's duty of care to the individual patient, whereas the stuff of EBM is necessarily statistical.

One might also see EBM as reinforcing the long-standing favoured position enjoyed by high-tech acute interventions at the expense of overall quality of care, for a patient who may not really require the high-tech acute intervention but who is pressured into it because treatment evidence is better. That is, some treatments may become the norm not because they are actually better, but because the evidence for them is better.[25] One survey of general practitioners uncovered the quirk that four out of their five preferred 'top' drugs issued from chance discoveries or personal belief rather than from clinical trials – penicillin, aspirin, corticosteroids and insulin, with cemetidine as the odd one out.[26] Chance can actually be a fine thing, although the brunt of this book has presented luck as problematic in medicine.

From the viewpoint of luck and randomness, EBM can likewise be construed as using randomness – in the randomized clinical trial – in order to defeat luck, particularly luck in antecedent circumstances. Because it is apparently unjust that whether or not patients obtain particular treatments should depend on 'postcode prescribing', on what treatments their local health authority recommends for funding, the objective is to defeat ill-luck through greater systematization.

Even committed advocates of EBM must acknowledge, however, that all health-care provision will never be evidence-based. It has been estimated that in only, at best, 20 per cent of cases is evidence from randomized clinical trials (RCTs) available.[27] In some of the cases where evidence exists, results of these RCTs are still difficult to extrapolate to daily practice. The traditional skills of a doctor, insofar as they represent an 'art' or a 'craft' rather than a 'social science', are not necessarily compatible with the skills required to interpret statistical evidence in meta-analyses.

Berg[28] acknowledges four dangerous aspects of protocols, which might well bear on the duties of a doctor. First of all, the growing interest in protocols strengthens the tendency to describe medical practice as a process of individual, formal-rational decisions, denying its social character. Secondly, protocols reinforce the illusion of the single answer. Thirdly, in protocols information and interventions that are difficult to make explicit or quantify are lost. Finally, Berg thinks that it is naïve to believe that protocols will not increase bureaucracy and will not put more external control on health-care practice. Protocols will make information accessible to third parties who can take advantage of the information, such as insurance companies. Stoop, Berg and Dinant express similar concerns.[29]

In the last section, I argued for what I regard as a more subtle outlook. It is impossible to defeat all the operations of luck and chance, and better to recognize their impact openly. Against the claim that it is irresponsible for policy-makers not to seek to act on maximal information, it might be regarded as equally irresponsible – and arrogant – not to recognize the limitations of information. This was the crux of my argument against Richard Brandt's position in chapter 3. Randomness as an allocation device, as I also argued in the previous section of this chapter, draws the fire of chance by recognizing it openly. Similarly, the communication process in properly informed consent, as I argued in chapters 4 and 5, forces patient and doctor alike to recognize risks, rather than skate over them in the fond hope that the outcome will be favourable.

Furthermore, there are grounds for believing that a rigid application of EBM will increase injustice by favouring groups who are already receiving a disproportionate share of resources and prejudicing the interests of those who are already disadvantaged.[30] There are a number of reasons for thinking that justice may sometimes collide with efficiency in the wider use of EBM.[31] Randomized clinical trials are easier to organize for acute conditions than for chronic ones, for younger patients than for elderly ones (although not for children), and for competent patients than for patients lacking mental capacity. In particular, because the large-scale trials underpinning EBM are expensive, they are more likely to be funded if they involve testing pharmaceuticals – funded by pharmaceutical companies. Palliative care, neonatal care and psychiatry are among the branches of medicine in which clinical trials are often either ethically debatable or difficult to compare in terms of results from a control and an experimental arm. It may be that these specialities are not innately disadvantaged; EBM may evolve beyond its initial concentration on drug-based therapies and acute medicine. But it does seem likely that they will be *prima facie* disadvantaged.[32]

A prime example is the long-simmering debate on whether beta-interferon for multiple sclerosis should be made available on the NHS, which has finally boiled down to a definite recommendation by NICE against routine prescription of the drug. Here we have a group of sufferers from a chronic rather than an acute condition, and a case in which the benefit derived is not thought to be proportionate to the cost, on the basis of QALYs (estimated variously at £81,000–£248,000 over five years). Luck-based inequality in 'postcode prescribing' has been eliminated, but only by substituting a 'very British fudge' whereby eligible patients must be entered in a monitoring exercise to receive the drug. By contrast, randomization was used in allocating beta-interferon when the drug was first made available for the treatment of multiple sclerosis in the United States, through development of a nationwide lottery involving a waiting list of 57,000 patients. Medical criteria were used initially to restrict eligibility for the lottery: patients had to be able to walk at least 100 yards and had to have the relapsing-remitting form of the disease. A tracking system guarded against attempts by wealthy patients to buy extra lottery tickets. 'Most of my patients are accepting the wait pretty well', commented one neurologist, 'because there is an element of fairness in a lottery.'[33]

Let us return to the fivefold typology of models introduced in the previous section on resource allocation at the clinical level:

- medical criteria: prognosis
- medical criteria: diagnosis
- social criteria: past merit
- social criteria: future merit
- randomized allocation.

This typology is also useful here, in this section on allocation of scarce resource at the public policy level. Evidence-based medicine is rooted in the first of our five criteria, medical (prognosis), and in the QALY methodology. But that method of decision-making, which is central to the UK National Institute for Clinical Excellence, also incorporates social factors, perhaps unwittingly. In particular, allocation by QALYs tends to favour the young over the elderly, since there are more future life-years to be gained by preferring young people over old. Whereas few governments have been willing to 'bite the bullet' and deny health care services to everyone over a certain age, the effect of using QALYs as the main tool of current resource allocation policy in the UK is just that.

The philosopher John Harris has drawn attention to this discriminatory aspect of QALYs,[34] but he has also defended another form of socially based allocation. Whereas QALYs centre on future 'merit', however, Harris's 'fair innings' argument represents an unusual kind of 'past desert' strategy. Generally 'past desert' models recommend awarding the scarce resource to those who have made particularly noteworthy, socially beneficial achievements in the past. Having had one's 'fair innings' means that one has had one's 'just deserts', and should *not* receive preference for treatment now.

Although on the 'macro' level people might well be uncomfortable with denying health care resources to everyone over a certain age, on the 'micro' level most people would probably find preferring the younger person perfectly acceptable. Harris effectively reverses the usual preferences. If there is only one dialysis machine or kidney available, and a choice must be made between giving it to a seventy-year-old or a twenty-year-old, the commonsense answer seems obvious enough. Harris, however, calls this commonsense preference an unacceptable form of ageism that contradicts respect for persons. The seventy-year-old's attachment to life may be just as great as that of the twenty-year-old. More generally, patients with short life expectancies may be as 'worthy' of receiving the scarce medical resource as those with longer expectancies.

Harris is actually willing to give *greater* weight to the desire for life in the patient with a shorter expectation of it, in this example:

Suppose I am told today that I have terminal cancer with only approximately six months or so to live, but I want to live until I die, or at least until I decide that life is no longer worth living. Suppose I then am involved in an accident and because my condition is known to my potential rescuers and there are not enough resources to treat all those who could be immediately saved I am marked among those who will not be helped. I am then the victim of a double tragedy and a double injustice. I am stricken first by cancer and the knowledge that I have only a short time to live and I'm then stricken again when I'm told that because of my first tragedy a second and more immediate one is to be visited upon me. Because I have once been unlucky I'm no longer worth saving.[35]

I find this argument from ill-luck quite compelling, but it is disappointing that Harris backtracks almost immediately by introducing an opposing argument, grounded in 'fair innings'. Whereas the 'anti-ageism' argument openly took the agent's subjective valuation of life as the criterion, the fair innings perspective sets a supposedly objective standard, the statistically average lifespan. (Harris should really divide the 'average' lifespan into male and female spans if he wants to avoid disadvantaging women, but this is not my main criticism.) Beyond this limit, set at seventy, the anti-ageism argument is not to trespass. No one over that age is to be allowed the scarce medical resource in preference to someone under that age, no matter how intense the older person's desire for life is or how disadvantaged their life has been so far.

Admittedly, desire to live is not the only factor to be considered. There is also the good of living beyond twenty, which the seventy-year-old has already enjoyed. In Robert Veatch's view, justice as fairness demands 'that persons be given an opportunity to have well-being over a lifetime equal to that of others. This means that infants, who have had no opportunity for well-being, would get a higher priority than older persons who have had many good years of life.'[36] But what if the years have not been good – if the person concerned has had a long run of ill-luck in antecedent circumstances? Surely Harris was originally right to draw our attention to the way in which being disadvantaged before, through prior ill-luck, is exacerbated by further ill-luck in denial of resources.

Because people in modern Western societies *do* live to an average of something like seventy says nothing at all about whether they *should* live to seventy, or more. To argue otherwise is a form of the naturalistic fallacy, and an attempt – like EBM – to avoid confronting ethical questions about justice in resource allocation by substituting supposedly objective criteria. In fact the preference for treating younger people over older people might merely be seen as a prejudice of our youth-mad culture. But youth is not a form of social merit.

Throughout this chapter I have been bucking the trend towards supposedly objective clinical indicators and away from confronting difficult ethical questions. My argument has been that the merit of randomization as a principle of allocation is twofold: it treats as equals everyone requiring treatment, and it forces us to look justifications for other ways of dividing people up squarely in the face. As in the beta-interferon example, however, I am willing to recognize some preliminary place for both medical and social criteria in policy-making, in selecting who may enter a lottery for a new treatment or be added to a waiting list. There the preliminary criterion was that, before being entered in the lottery to receive the drug, the patient should have the remitting-relapsing form of multiple sclerosis and should be able to walk 100 yards. Similarly, there may be some social criteria that ought to be invoked prior to allocating the scarce resource by random means among those who qualify. Merely because social criteria were heavily discredited by the Seattle 'God' Committee does not mean that they have no place whatsoever. Most medical ethicists recognize the unassailability of anti-social worth arguments; debate now centres on whether exceptions are ever justified.[37] Beauchamp and Childress, for example, limit their advocacy of random allocation by allowing some role for social worth 'in exceptional cases involving persons of critical social importance'.[38] Their argument is tinged with an efficiency-centred consequentialism, however: although we cannot determine social worth in ordinary cases, they claim, in exceptional cases we can judge it accurately enough to produce more value than if social worth criteria were not applied.

My argument is more deontological: we should depart from random allocation in cases where duties rather than desert hold sway. The effect of this exception will be to prefer those who have immediate duties towards dependants, either children or elderly parents. One might view this as a form of ill-luck in antecedent circumstances, whereas Harris, for example, views having children as a 'good' which some privileged souls possess and other less fortunate individuals do not enjoy. (He even goes on to suggest that a resource allocation policy favouring parents of young children might lead people to 'acquire' children in order to benefit from 'a relatively cheap form of insurance against a low-priority rating in the rescue stakes'.[39]) Although also a utilitarian, Jonathan Glover contests this point:

Refusal to depart from random choice when knowledge about ... dependants is available is to place no value on avoiding the additional misery caused to the children if the mother is not the one saved...A large part of the case against interventionism is the undesirability of creating a two-tier system, saying that we value some people more than others. This seems obviously objectionable if our preference is based on the belief that one of the people is nicer, more intelligent, or morally superior to the other person. But the objection loses a lot of its force when the preference is justified by citing the interests of dependants rather than the merits of the person selected.[40]

Mothers are particularly disadvantaged – rather than favoured, as Harris claims – by the economic costs of having children, in terms of lost earnings during childbearing and child-rearing years, along with diminished pension and seniority rights.[41] Fathers of dependent children are a more difficult issue, since they might claim to be equally bound by duty – the traditional duty to provide. However, this particular responsibility has in fact been a source of privilege – through the trade union policy of the family wage, for instance, which systematically rewarded male workers and preserved income differentials between men and women.[42] In order to avoid the accumulation of further advantage for those already fortunate in their antecedent circumstances – for the reason feared by Glover and Harris alike, the avoidance of a two-tier system – I would view fathers of dependent children as having no claim to special treatment unless the children live with them (if the parents are separated) or unless they do at least half of the actual child care (if the parents are together).

The exception to randomness for mothers and some fathers of dependent children does not threaten the general structure of my argument in favour of randomness as an allocation device at both the macro and the micro levels. No judgement is being made of these parents' social worth, prognosis or diagnosis. Instead, we are attempting to avoid additional ill-luck for the children of the affected parent, in the manner described by Glover (or for the elderly parent who loses the primary carer). It seems unlikely that clinicians would feel remorse or regret at having preferred a primary carer over someone who had no duties towards dependants, even if the chosen patient did not recover and the scarce resource was 'wasted'. As with informed consent, the way out of the dilemmas of moral luck is to ensure that the procedure is as fair as possible, regardless of how the outcome turns out.

It may well occasion regret if, in the course of following a policy of randomization, a ninety-year-old who satisfies the preliminary medical criteria and is entered into a lottery or waiting list 'wins out' over a twenty-year-old. That might well be deeply sad, but it would not necessarily be unjust.[43] Nor would it be an instance of moral luck. Provided that moral agents make their decisions about resource allocation according to the right principle – and I argue that randomization is generally the right principle – they can satisfy Nagel's maxim, I think, however things actually turn out. That is, they have no reason to modify whatever decision they would have taken in light of their knowledge of subsequent events.

7

Reproductive Ethics: What Risks Can Women be Asked to Bear?

Risk, contract and 'surrogacy'

There are interesting moral luck questions in 'surrogacy': for example, the question of whether a 'surrogate' can rightfully bind herself to deliver up the child, given that she cannot know in advance what her future emotional response will be to pregnancy and childbirth.[1] But although I am intrigued by the parallel with Gauguin's uncertainty as to whether he would discover the qualities of a great painter in himself, once he had made his choice, moral luck in outcome or character will not be my primary focus in this part of the chapter. Instead I want to think about risk and contract.

In my 1997 book *Property, Women and Politics*, I drew attention to the question of what happens if 'surrogacy' goes wrong, arguing that we ought to be more concerned with giving contract mothers protection in the event of miscarriage or the birth of a severely disabled child. In this chapter I want to argue, similarly, that a risk-oriented argument, one focusing on outcome luck, supports partial legalization of contract motherhood – but only if the object of the contract is the mother's pain and suffering rather than the baby. At the beginning of the discussion, however, I also want to return to the conclusions of chapter 4 on informed consent, which suggests a tension with my argument about 'surrogacy' and contract. If a contract mother has given her consent, as expressed in a contract, does that mean that she now bears all responsibility for ill-luck in outcomes?

A related but different question is whether paying a woman to bear certain risks, and her acceptance of payment on that basis, absolves other parties, including the state, of responsibility if things go wrong. The answer is clearly no. Employment law is predicated on the premise that employers cannot absolve themselves of all risk when workers agree to work for them; nor can the state shake off its responsibilities to provide regulation of employers and benefits for those who lose their health or jobs. And there are some risks that we simply do not allow people to assume, no matter how much they are paid for them: we do not allow people to sell a kidney, for example.[2] Although 'surrogacy' poses some unique problems, the point I want to make clear at the outset is that we do not necessarily allow all responsibility to be borne solely by one party even where that party has accepted payment to carry some of the responsibility. The answer to the question 'what risks can women be asked to bear?' will not be simply 'those that they are paid to bear'. On the other hand, I will not accept as a knock-down argument the claim that the risks of pregnancy should not be run for money.

Another preliminary question involves terminology. The use of the term 'surrogate' implies that the birth mother is not the real mother. Although some US jurisdictions do view the genetic mother as the legal mother – in cases where the birth mother is not the genetic mother – English law regards the birth mother as the legal mother, on the principle *mater est quam gestatio demonstrat*, and so do I. It is only by discounting women's labour in childbirth that the birth mother can be seen as a 'surrogate'. Another way of putting this objection is to say that, 'in truth, the surrogate is a surrogate for maternity, not motherhood',[3] although I am less happy with that formulation because it implies that motherhood is 'merely' biological.

However, there are problems in using the term 'contract' mother where no legally binding contract can be involved, in jurisdictions such as the UK. 'Gestational' mother is sometimes used in the literature, but that terminology again tends to imply that there is also another mother, the 'genetic' mother, whose claims may be greater than those of the gestational mother (again, where the genetic mother is not the gestational mother). Awkward as it is, I have therefore chosen to use 'surrogate' throughout in inverted commas. The awkwardness will perhaps serve a function in reminding readers continually that it is wrong to call a 'surrogate' mother a surrogate mother. My apologies to readers who do not need reminding.

Finally, I shall also be avoiding the confusing terms 'full' and 'partial' surrogacy. As Robert Lee and Derek Morgan rightly remark, 'surrogacy' is always 'full' for the 'surrogate': 'The descriptions "full" and "partial" surrogacy which have more recently entered the lexicons of assisted conception are really misnomers: it is not the surrogacy that is partial, it is the contribution of the commissioning couple that genetically is partial or full.'[4] Both 'surrogacy' and its subdivisions 'full' and 'partial' are value-laden: they already prejudge the argument about who is the real parent in favour of the genetic parent(s) rather than the birth mother. These terms both demonstrate and create an imbalance in the power relationship between commissioning couple and 'surrogate' mother. We need to think about that from the outset, too, in deciding what risks women can be asked to bear.

I begin with a case study in which contract apparently failed to protect the pregnant woman from possible exploitation by the commissioning couple. I then develop the study further in light of three possible approaches to risk minimization and legalization, and finally compare my conclusions with the recommendations made in the UK Brazier Committee report of 1998, which came down against legalization of 'surrogacy' contracts.

> The legal wrangle involving a British woman carrying surrogate twins for an American couple took another twist yesterday when a new set of prospective parents offered to take on the babies after they are born.
>
> Helen Beasley, 26, is suing Charles Wheeler and Martha Berman for allegedly backing out of the £14,000 deal when they discovered she was carrying twins.
>
> Ms Beasley, who claims the couple from San Francisco abandoned her when she refused to abort one of the foetuses, has filed lawsuits in the San Diego superior court, claiming breach of contract and misrepresentation, and demanding unspecified damages for medical costs and emotional suffering.
>
> Dianne Michelsen, attorney for Mr Wheeler and Ms Berman, yesterday announced that they had found another set of prospective parents for the children.
>
> 'This family has passed the necessary medical, emotional and psychological screenings to be approved by their state regulatory agency,' Ms Michelsen said.
>
> However, Ms Beasley's lawyer, Theresa Erickson, said that her client wanted a say in who the adoptive parents should be and did not accept the couple proposed by Mr Wheeler and Ms Berman. Ms Erickson said that Ms Beasley had found a suitable couple three months earlier but an agreement fell through when Mr Wheeler and Ms Berman demanded a 'larger sum of money' for relinquishing their parental rights.
>
> Appearing on American television, Ms Erickson said the legal secretary from Shrewsbury in Shropshire was also claiming compensation for her surrogacy.

'She has lost her job in England and she has nothing here except for what people are giving her,' the lawyer said.

Ms Beasley, who has a nine-year-old son, made contact with the couple, who are both San Francisco lawyers, via the internet. They agreed to pay her £14,000 and made an initial payment of £700, according to Ms Erickson.

She underwent in vitro fertilisation at the Zouves fertility centre in Daly City, California, a month later using Mr Wheeler's sperm and eggs from a donor.

Under the terms of the contract Ms Beasley agreed to abort additional foetuses if more than one egg was fertilised.

But she claims they verbally agreed that any decision would be made before the 12th week of the pregnancy, only to be told at the end of the 13th week that the couple wished for the abortion to take place.

Ms Beasley said she would not consider aborting one of the foetuses because her pregnancy was too far gone and the procedure could risk the life of the other twin.

'They don't want two babies and although we did have it in the contract that if there were multiples we would reduce, they left it too late in arranging an appointment to reduce them.

'I thought I just couldn't do it. There is a risk to the other baby as well. If you abort one the risk of miscarriage is high and you could lose both of them.'[5]

This case also illustrates ill-luck in outcomes – only if, like the commissioning parents, one views twins as a form of ill-luck – but my discussion will focus more on risk than luck. What sorts of risk are at issue here? Apart from the risks of signing a contract with two American lawyers, the *medical risks* to the 'surrogate' and foetus(es) might include the following.

- *The risks of undergoing IVF.* Although Ms Beasley appears to be fertile (or was at the time her son was born) the couple have required her to undergo IVF, using the man's sperm but not the woman's oocytes. (It is not entirely clear why donor oocytes were used: the usual rationale for IVF would be that the commissioning couple want the baby to contain both their genetic material.) If the pregnancy had been created through simple donor insemination (DI), Ms Beasley would have been spared the possibly carcinogenic effects of superovulation, and the anaesthetic and surgical risks of egg extraction, together with the risks involved in implantation of two or more embryos (as has clearly occurred in this case). Some jurisdictions, particularly in the Nordic countries, now forbid implanting more than one embryo after IVF because of the risks to the woman and foetus. In the UK the Human Fertilisation and Embryology Authority recently passed regulations permitting no more than two embryos to be implanted. In the USA implantation of more than two embryos is still routine, although usually no more than four.[6] Commercial 'surrogacy' agencies and private IVF centres have an interest, of course, in higher success rates from implanting multiple embryos. The question of whether it is permissible for them to impose the attendant risks on women is muddied by women's interest in undergoing as few treatment cycles as possible. Although there was no physiological need for Ms Beasley to undergo IVF rather than simple DI – indeed, some IVF specialists maintain that use of the procedure for a fertile woman is an unjustified use of resources and an illicit imposition of risks – commercial 'surrogacy' arrangements often specify IVF because the 'surrogate' is believed to be more willing to give up the baby if it is not genetically related to her.[7]

- *Risk to the second foetus* in attempting to abort the first.[8]
- *Risk to the pregnant woman of undergoing an abortion* at a comparatively advanced stage of pregnancy.
- *Risk of continuing the pregnancy and undergoing a twin delivery*, which is more likely to require a Caesarean section, involving a 20–45 per cent risk of infection and a maternal death rate for emergency Caesareans of 25.2 per 100,000 births (as against a figure of 1.8 for vaginal deliveries).[9]
- In other cases than this, *more general risks such as ectopic pregnancy* and other sequelae of pregnancy. For example, one of the women interviewed in Helena Ragone's analysis of the motivations of 'surrogate' mothers nearly bled to death in an ectopic 'surrogate' pregnancy,[10] although even 'surrogates' who have suffered difficult pregnancies or deliveries typically claim to have babies easily – perhaps not least because that is part of what the US agencies who pay them are looking for.

In addition there are *'social' risks* for the 'surrogate', including the following.

- *The possibility that commissioning parents will refuse to take custody* of a child who is surplus to requirements, as in this case, or otherwise not to their liking (e.g., born with a disability, or of the 'wrong' sex).

- *Possible strain on other relationships.* For example, husbands of 'surrogates' are routinely required to sign a form promising to abstain from sex until the 'surrogate' has conceived by the contracting man and the pregnancy has been confirmed.[11] Ms Beasley is unmarried, but she broke off her job and other relationships in the UK in order to undergo IVF and 'surrogate' pregnancy in the USA.
- *Financial risks.* Ms Beasley is now unemployed and has nothing to show for her labour in undergoing IVF and the early stages of pregnancy except a small initial payment, which is not enough for her to live on. She probably also lacks medical insurance. If the twins are not adopted, she bears the financial responsibility for them until they reach the age of majority.
- *Family dysfunction.* Although the then UK Secretary for Health, Kenneth Clarke, said in 1985 that there were few or no ethical problems with 'surrogacy' arrangements between sisters, I myself know of a UK case in which a sister-in-law agreed verbally to bear a child for an infertile couple, but then retracted her agreement to surrender the child. The ensuing difficulties caused severe family problems for a very long time. In another UK case Lori Jasso, who had four young children, was asked by her eldest sister to carry a child for her. Eight years after the birth of the baby, Tiana, she had not been allowed to see the child since the elder sister took her away at birth. As Jasso said, 'I felt raped by sisterly love.'[12]

The risks for the commissioning couple are less obvious except for the principal 'weapon' in the 'surrogate's' armoury:

- *The 'surrogate' may refuse to deliver the child.* In this case, however, the reverse problem has occurred: Ms Beasley wants to hand over not one but two children. Although the commissioning couple refuse to take custody of twins, they still demand a substantial sum to give up their 'parental rights' to choose who should adopt the babies.[13] It was claimed that they were also prepared to surrender the twins to 'the highest bidder' for £55,000. If this is true, then their financial risks, at least, are minimal: indeed, one might say they enjoyed 'a handsome return'.[14]

There are at least three possible approaches to dealing with these sorts of risks. The first is to say that the decision about whether a woman should be asked to bear them should be pre-empted by legislation.

This approach can in turn be subdivided into legislating against commercial contract motherhood versus leaving private arrangements between 'consenting' individuals unregulated. This is roughly the approach taken by UK law since the Warnock Committee's recommendations, with the ensuing passage of the Surrogacy Arrangements Act 1985 and the Human Fertilisation and Embryology Act 1990. Although an attempt in the House of Lords failed to make all aspects of 'surrogacy' criminal, including private non-commercial arrangements, agencies may be criminally prosecuted under the 1985 Act from advertising for 'surrogate' mothers, negotiating 'surrogacy' arrangements on a for-profit basis, or making anything that may be construed as 'a promise or understanding that payment will or may be made to the ['surrogate' mother] or for her benefit' (s1(4)). 'Surrogacy' contracts are legally unenforceable (s36 of the HFE Act), although both the 'surrogate' and the commissioning couple are exempt from criminal prosecution. Interestingly, the reasoning was to protect not the 'surrogate' but the possible child – from having a parent who was 'subject to the taint of criminality'.[15]

The second approach views the first as unacceptably paternalistic. If other people can be asked to bear risks for an appropriate reward in cash – deep-sea divers, riveters on high-rise tower blocks – then so can contract mothers. This approach, taken by John Harris[16] and also by some feminist writers,[17] is roughly the position in many US states, where 'surrogacy' contracts are legally enforceable and commercial 'surrogate' agencies operate freely.[18] The Internet muddies the difference between the two jurisdictions – as in this case, where a woman from a country in which a 'surrogacy' contract would be unenforceable has contracted with nationals of a jurisdiction that does allow commercial 'surrogacy', and in which the contract is enforceable.

A third approach, the one that I developed in *Property, Women and Politics*, agrees with the second that there is a role for contract in 'surrogacy', but limits it to contracting for the women's labour, pain and suffering in pregnancy and childbirth. Contract should not extend to the right or duty to contract away the baby. I share the concern of the first approach for protecting women from exploitation, but I believe that is done more effectively through allowing contract some role. That does not necessarily mean unrestricted freedom of contract: as Joan Mahoney has pointed out, restrictions on absolute freedom of contract are inevitable and are accepted under anything but barefaced capitalism. Precluding gestational mothers from contracting away their babies no more hampers their economic autonomy than does any other form of employment protection.[19] With the globalization of capitalism, and of the new reproductive technologies – as illustrated particularly vividly in the case study, although ongoing over the past decade[20] – it becomes harder but all the more necessary to impose some such restrictions.

Ms Beasley is trying to use the contract she drew up with the commissioning parents to protect herself against risk (particularly the risks in late abortion, since she appears to be willing to undergo the risks of twin pregnancy and childbirth). In the UK she would not have any such protection if the commissioning parents decided to withdraw from an informal arrangement. Ms Beasley may or may not win her case in the San Diego courts, but the point is that she can bring a case in the first place, because the contract is enforceable on both sides. This particular contract may not have been drafted in such a way as to protect her sufficiently, but the solution is to ensure that contracts do protect 'surrogates' by binding the commissioning couple to compensate the woman for her lost employment, labour and suffering – all of which Ms Beasley is claiming – regardless of whether the babies meet their specifications. These are uncompensated risks under the usual 'surrogacy' contracts, which specify that the baby must be transferred, in a form acceptable to the contracting couple – in this case the only acceptable form being 'baby' rather than 'babies' – before the gestational mother's risk-taking is compensated. Similarly, when the foetus spontaneously aborts, is stillborn, or is born with a severe disability, a 'surrogacy' contract needs to protect the gestational mother.[21]

Although this proposal may seem far-fetched, it is actually nothing like as counter-intuitive as selling babies, which is what current 'surrogacy' contracts amount to. The gestational mother can sell *only* her labour; that is all she has to sell, short of allowing trafficking in children. In the *Anna J.* case,[22] the judge in fact recognized that what the gestational mother was selling was her pain and suffering in pregnancy and labour. Although that case went against the mother, because the genetic parents were seen as having prior custody rights over the baby by sheer virtue of *being* the genetic parents, it provides legal backing for my proposal. Essentially my argument is that labour in childbirth *is* labour, although that is rarely recognized.[23] Labour, on a Lockean account, confers a property right.

Rather than openly banning 'surrogacy', the third approach could concentrate on overturning existing legal presumptions that favour men, such as the assumption of genetically conferred custody rights, and on ensuring that 'surrogacy' contracts are worded so stringently as to eliminate exploitation of women. Non-liberal feminists have tended to see the source of exploitation in the economic imbalance between the contracting parents and the gestational mother, and in the comparatively low level of payment for 'surrogacy'. Both factors are present in the case above, but what is more important is to ensure that labour in childbirth is viewed as women's property. The effect of the distinction between labour and baby, combined with the Lockean assertion that women own their labour, is to curtail women's propertylessness in their own labour, which 'surrogacy' arrangements could otherwise exacerbate. A second effect is to ensure that women are fully compensated for all the risks they undergo in pregnancy and childbirth, rather than compensated for handing over the baby. 'Surrogacy' is often viewed as merely renting out a womb,[24] and the 'surrogate' mother has been described in at least one court of law as being like a foster-mother who cares for the child when the 'true parents' are temporarily unavailable.[25] But this is radically to underestimate what women do, and the risks they endure, in pregnancy and childbirth. For this reason parallels with prostitution, as renting out one's body, also fail, whether made by feminists such as Carole Pateman[26] or by libertarian utilitarians such as John Harris.

If the 'surrogacy' contract is for the woman's labour and risk-taking in pregnancy and childbirth, the birth mother will be able to enforce a claim against the commissioning father or couple even if the child is not to the their liking – if there are too many children, if the child is stillborn or disabled, if the child is of the 'wrong' sex. If the contract is for pregnancy *or* childbirth, she can claim protection against the risk of miscarriage.[27] She has none of these protections if 'surrogacy' contracts are void in law, as advocates of the first position would prefer. Whether or not commissioning couples would accept a contract framed in these terms is, as the saying goes, not my problem. Since in the USA, at least, couples such as the one in the case study have effectively been buying babies with impunity for some time, they can hardly claim the moral high ground. More pragmatically, I imagine that there would still be some 'takers' among commissioning couples for a contract limited to the gestational mother's labour, rather than a property in or custody of the baby. In many cases, such as the one above, the gestational mother will wish to have the baby (or babies) adopted if the commissioning parents reject it (or them), or if other difficulties arise in the relationship with the commissioning couple. This is actually close to the adoption model of 'surrogacy', which many commentators feel is the only morally admissible one.[28] The contract can rightfully be only for the 'surrogate's' labour in pregnancy and childbirth, and the subsequent custody of the child is best left to the adoption mechanisms (or, in the UK, to the 'parental order' mechanism under s30 of the Human Fertilisation and Embryology Act 1990). Many 'surrogate' mothers will still undertake their pregnancies in the expectation of surrendering the child to the commissioning couple, even if that is not specified in the contract; the mechanism for doing so will then be adoption rather than contract. Adoption proceedings are required to take the best interests of the child into account, which may still discriminate against 'surrogate' mothers, who typically cannot offer the child as financially cushioned an existence as the commissioning couple. But at least adoption does consider the child's interests, whereas a contract for transfer of a baby treats the baby simply as an object.

One difficulty I do have to face in proposing that contracts should not specify transfer of the baby is whether gestational mothers themselves would accept a 'surrogacy' contract along what they might see as hard-nosed lines. Helena Ragone's survey of American 'surrogates' found that they generally saw what they were doing in relational terms, even if it was in fact governed by contract: as giving a gift to someone needier than themselves, rather than as selling a service to someone who is positioned to exploit them.[29] This is not altogether surprising, since the advertisements for commercial US 'surrogacy' programmes are saturated with the language of gift ('give the gift of life' winning handily over most of the other clichés).[30] Although 'surrogates' sometimes mention money, they frequently protest that no one would become pregnant for money alone – actually because 'it isn't enough', a rather harder-headed response than one might expect.[31]

Money, however, removes the personal element from the 'relationship' with the commissioning couple. Ragone found that 'surrogates' are rather cynically encouraged by agencies to identify completely with the couple receiving the baby ('they are going to be as pregnant as you are');[32] some also feel that they are atoning for a previous adoption or abortion. (It is admittedly speculative, but perhaps Ms Beasley is 'atoning' for having become pregnant at sixteen or seventeen, as she must have been if, at the age of twenty-six she has a nine-year-old son.) Ragone's research also uncovered the practice of many commercial 'surrogacy' agencies in employing psychologists and counsellors whose function is to redefine and reinforce the notion of family ('extended' to encompass the 'surrogate' temporarily, but ratified as primarily the commissioning husband and wife).[33] The 'surrogate' is continually fed the messages that she is helping to create and maintain a traditional family for the commissioning couple, despite the rather unorthodox means being used to create it.

However, 'surrogates' are also deliberately misled by commissioning couples and commercial agencies into believing that the relationship with the contracting couple is something more than instrumental. Normally couples terminate the 'relationship' as soon as the baby is born, often to the 'surrogate's' great distress.[34] ('I felt they had been my friends, but after they got what they wanted, they weren't.')[35] The balance of power, Ragone found, lay firmly with the commissioning couple, who were after all paying the agency, and the 'surrogate' through the agency.[36] This imbalance is accentuated by the typical class profile of 'surrogates': in Ragone's survey the majority were working-class women with only a high-school education, whereas commissioning couples typically came from a higher social stratum.[37] Since the only 'leverage' of the 'surrogate' is to keep the child, it might even be that a more open form of contract of the form I suggest would reduce the angry reactions of disappointed contract mothers who have no other way of 'getting back' at commissioning couples when the 'relationship' breaks down than refusing to surrender the child.

Elizabeth Anderson has noted that this non-economic motivation renders contracting mothers ripe for exploitation. Indeed, she argues, that kind of exploitation is going on, whatever the economic rewards, when one party operates with norms based on commodity exchange while the other sees what she is doing as altruistic.[38] Here is another form of risk, a non-medical variant, and another sort of moral luck: it is a form of ill-luck in outcomes when a woman discovers that the couple whom she thought she was helping out of altruism actually view the transaction as purely commercial. That discovery also poses a risk to the woman's selfhood as a moral agent: she thought that her motivations had to do with being a good person, but those motivations were discounted by the commissioning couple. Another advantage of the third approach, then, would be to bring each side's understanding of whether this is a commercial transaction or an act of supererogatory selflessness out into the open.

The UK's Brazier Committee did consider the third approach,[39] but ultimately decided to continue with something more like the first. Case law had in fact taken something more like the third approach: for example, the 1987 decision in *Re an Adoption Application (Sur-*

rogacy) in which Lacey J. held that payments made to a 'surrogate' were for her time and inconvenience, not for transfer of the baby. Implicitly rejecting that parallel as specious, the Brazier Committee report recommended that payment to 'surrogates' should cover no more than fully documented expenses and that additional payments should be prohibited to prevent the commercialization of 'surrogacy'. Contracts for 'surrogacy' should remain unenforceable, and the existing bans on advertising and for-profit arrangements should continue. Although the Brazier Committee was concerned to protect the welfare of the child and of the 'surrogate', it was heavily influenced by the view that paid 'surrogacy' is indistinguishable from selling children. As Brazier has written elsewhere, although it may be argued that an infertile couple are not buying a baby when they hire a 'surrogate', 'that argument is specious. If in the UK we wish to sustain objections to trade in babies, payments to surrogates should continue to be outlawed, and continuing payments to gamete donors must be, at least, a cause for concern.'[40]

As Lee and Morgan note, my third approach also drives a wedge between hiring a 'surrogate' and buying a baby, which must be a good thing. I think it is an illegitimate jump in both logic and policy to say that all payments to 'surrogates' must be outlawed if we wish to sustain objections to trade in babies, although I fully accept those objections. Most particularly for the present purpose, I am concerned that the Brazier formulations fail to protect 'surrogates' from risk. Other writers, such as Michael Freeman, have also criticized the Brazier Committee on similar grounds: 'Brazier is too readily dismissive of the distinction between payment for the purchase of a child and payment for a potentially risky, time-consuming and uncomfortable service.'[41] While I feel that 'uncomfortable' as a description of labour in childbirth is a front-running contender for the understatement of the millennium prize, I agree with the rest of Freeman's analysis, although not with its primarily consequentialist foundations.

The language of 'exploitation' was prominent in the original Warnock Committee report:

> Even in compelling medical circumstances the danger of exploitation of one human being by another appears to the majority of us to far outweigh the potential benefits in almost every case.[42]

Although the Brazier Committee also claimed to be concerned about possible exploitation of the 'surrogate', the language of the consultation document and the final findings frequently seem to view the 'surrogate' as exploiter rather than exploited. The terms of reference for the review began with the question 'whether payments, including expenses, to surrogate mothers should continue to be allowed, and if so on what basis.'[43] Nevertheless, the terms of the consultation invited an alternative solution such as my third approach:

> We have specifically asked the review team to consider the issue within the context that surrogacy should not be commercialised and that any woman who has a baby as part of a surrogacy arrangement should not be compelled to give it up if she changes her mind. We also want to know whether there is, realistically, any practical way in which surrogacy arrangements could or should be regulated and if so how.[44]

While the Warnock Committee was concerned to prevent exploitation, it failed to explore the ways in which exploitation can still occur even if 'surrogacy' contracts are not enforceable in law. In this respect it was as one with many other writers on 'surrogacy': Martha Field, for example, argues in favour of non-enforcement on the grounds of women's autonomy:

> Non-enforcement allows women to enter into these arrangements and to go through with them on whatever terms they choose ... All non-enforcement does is to protect the woman who herself decides that she does not want to go through with the arrangement after all.[45]

But non-enforcement also protects the couple who do not want to go through with the arrangement. Most of the power is already on their side: the very language in which the 'surrogacy' debate is conducted favours them, as I noted at the beginning. Now that professional bodies such as the British Medical Association have dropped their opposition to surrogacy,[46] and now that such arrangements are increasingly made internationally, over the Internet, there are fewer and fewer protections for the 'surrogate'. It seems to me that the Brazier Committee missed an important chance to protect 'surrogates' against the increasing risks they run.

The principle of non-enforcement is right in one important sense: the mother should not be forced to hand over the baby. The principle of enforceable contracts is correct in a different sense: the risks are loaded so heavily against the 'surrogate' mother that it will take a partially enforceable contract to protect her. That contract should be limited to the labour the 'surrogate' undergoes in pregnancy and childbirth, as well as in IVF (if applicable). I have argued elsewhere that contract, in a Hegelian sense, requires recognition of the other party in a relationship.[47] Although Ms Beasley's contract was imperfect, it has got her some recognition, and some chance of success in the courts. The language of 'surrogacy', 'partial' and 'full', is so loaded against the recognition of the woman undergoing pregnancy and childbirth as the real mother that the only way to redress the balance and see through the blind spot is through a revised and improved form of contract that forces the commissioning parties to recognize the 'surrogate' as an agent, not just as a womb for rent.

Therapeutic and human cloning

As with 'surrogacy', an approach focusing on what risks women can rightfully be asked to bear produces unconventional results in relation to therapeutic and human cloning, because it is a surprisingly unconventional way of considering the problem. The dominant discourse in cloning has concerned the identity of the clone (for reproductive human cloning) and/or of the embryo (for therapeutic cloning). When a distinction is made between therapeutic and human cloning, it is usually on the basis that reproductive cloning is offensive to human dignity because it denies the agency, autonomy and individuality of the clone. For example, the European Parliament resolution against cloning finds reproductive cloning deplorable because 'each individual has a right to his or her own genetic identity.'[48] This argument is easy meat to philosophers such as John Harris, who points out that no one doubts the agency, individuality and autonomy of each member of a pair of twins.[49]

Those who also oppose therapeutic cloning typically base their arguments on the moral status of the embryo: for example, in Germany all forms of embryo research are forbidden under the provisions of the *Embryonenschutzgesetz*, because use of the embryo at blastocyst stage 'kills' it – although research using existing stem cell lines imported from elsewhere is rather hypocritically permitted. In the UK, by contrast, recent legislation permits research on embryos up to fourteen days old not only for fertility-related purposes, as in the original Human Fertilisation and Embryology Act, but also for other research aims such as the development of stem cell lines. In the USA a compromise detested by all parties has been announced by President Bush, forbidding federal funds for future stem cell research involving the creation of embryos but permitting the use of stem cell lines created before 9 August 2001.[50] Whatever the considerable differences in legislation, all these approaches are concerned primarily with the moral status of the embryo. That is where the moral questions lie, in the dominant discourse; both opponents and proponents of stem cell research agree on that much. In both reproductive and therapeutic cloning, the focus is on the 'product' (the clone) or the 'raw material' (the embryo), but not on 'the worker' (the women who undergo superovulation and egg extraction to provide oocytes for enucleated eggs or who serve as 'surrogates').

To the extent that a feminist discourse appears in the literature, it comes, ironically, from proponents of cloning, who 'are seeking to appropriate the language of reproductive rights and freedom of choice to support their case'.[51] With few exceptions,[52] little is said about the risks to women that these procedures entail.

1   Both therapeutic and human cloning involve the enucleated egg technique that produced Dolly the sheep, but it took 267 'surrogate' ewes to produce Dolly. It might well take a comparable number of 'surrogate' mothers to produce one human clone.
2   Animal clones are much larger than average on birth. It has been estimated that a clone human baby would weigh fifteen pounds. Clearly the pain and suffering to the woman in childbirth would be immense. There would also be heightened risks of Caesarean section (see the risk figures for Caesareans above) and other complications of pregnancy and childbirth.
3   Animal clones suffer from a frighteningly high proportion of abnormalities, thought to result from bypassing the normal cell-division processes that weed out abnormal embryos as early miscarriages. As the Canadian bioethicist Laura Shanner remarks in her report to the Canadian health commission:

> Massive malformations in non-human animal offspring conceived by SCNT (somatic cell nuclear transfer) cloning should not be surprising in light of the known tendency toward spontaneous mutations in cell division. After many generations, genetic mistakes are likely to accumulate in somatic cells. For example, an apparently healthy epithelial cell may carry devastating but unexpressed errors in the genetic coding for, say, heart tissue. Attempting to derive transplantable cardiac cells from that apparently healthy epithelial cell would likely fail. Minor anomalies in unexpressed genes may even create new

rejection problems, thus undermining the proposed advantage of cloned stem cell cultures over tissue or organ transplants.[53]

Very recent research makes it uncertain whether the malfunctioning gene causing misexpression of the protein that produces these abnormalities exists in primates.[54] Until this question is resolved, we must take into account the high probability of a woman's giving birth to a baby who dies within a few days of gross abnormalities.

4   If the ultimate purpose of creating stem cell lines is to create replacement organs, we need to take into account the need for a 'host' – or hostess, in this case. Creating a replacement liver, for example, is not possible *in vitro*, although liver tissue might thrive. What would probably be required would be the transfer of primordial organs to a womb, human or otherwise.

5   The risks to women of ovum donation include the carcinogenic effects of superovulation and the risks of egg extraction under anaesthetic. Given that some IVF clinics routinely 'harvest' as many as seventy eggs,[55] it can readily be seen how unnatural these procedures are, and what possible side effects may arise. Although it is often said that women undergo no additional risk in embryo extraction to that which they would already be undergoing voluntarily in the course of IVF treatment, this argument ignores the ways in which women may be pressured to consent to higher regimes of ovarian stimulation than would be necessary to obtain three or four embryos to implant, and to further uses of 'surplus' embryos. Practices such as egg-sharing are increasingly allowed by the UK regulatory authority, the Human Fertilisation and Embryology Authority, and accepted as ethically unproblematic by many clinicians,[56] despite moral arguments against them that could and should be made on the basis of pressure on vulnerable women. If consent is to be obtained from women undergoing IVF, it needs to be for all the possible uses to which the 'surplus' embryos may be put, now and in the future. Furthermore, the creation of an immortal cell line from the 'surplus' embryos that a couple have created through IVF may seem a cruel mockery of their previous infertility. Ovum donation suffers from similar difficulties, since it is usually motivated by the altruistic desire to help other infertile couples.[57] How many women will wish to undergo the rigours of ovum donation in order to help biotechnology companies at worst, or vaguely specified 'research' at best?

The combination of these risks to living ovum donors is so great that Shanner believes the least objectionable course would be using cadaveric ovary donors.

6   Increasingly the conventional literature on stem cells seems to be turning towards advances in somatic cell technology or partheno-genesis as a way of bypassing ethical debates. The argument here is that no embryos or foetuses are involved, and therefore there are no ethical issues.[58] But somatic cells are not fully totipotent, and cannot be expected to yield as satisfactory stem cell lines as embryos or foetuses. It will therefore take many more enucleated eggs to produce one stem cell line from somatic cells than it would to produce a line from embryonic or foetal cells. In my view these developments may be more rather than less unethical, if they require larger numbers of eggs to be donated from women who are in a vulnerable position to act as egg donors or 'surrogate' mothers than would be the case if embryonic stem cells were used and if the attrition rate for embryonic stem cells is lower, as it appears to be. In addition, it is highly likely that more cell lines would be needed, since somatic cells are more specialized. Taken together, both these developments require more oocytes, and that means more risk to ovum donors. Whereas many proponents of stem cell research argue that surplus eggs from IVF are now sufficient,[59] the situation would alter if somatic cells were pre-ferred, and if there is to be a real increase in the number of cell lines above the current comparatively lower number. That argument seems doubtful even now: leading IVF clinicians in the UK have executed an about-face on stem cell research because there is already a shortage of donor eggs, which they fear will worsen if eggs are needed for therapeutic cloning.

Why are these risks so little known? Why has the debate over both human and therapeutic cloning turned almost exclusively on the status of the embryo? Just as in the abortion debate, which has turned on the moral status of the foetus, women's labour in pregnancy and childbirth is not recognized in the 'cloning wars'. It might even be argued that feminists have contributed to the problem, by agreeing to direct most of their fire to the question of whether the foetus has a moral personality. Even those few proponents of abortion who refuse to argue along the lines of the status of the foetus – such as Judith Jarvis Thomson – present what women do as merely *housing* the baby.[60] This is to ignore what women do in childbirth, and the additional and even riskier tasks they will be asked to undergo in the cloning technologies. The question of exploitation of women, as 'surrogates' or ovum donors, is typically brushed aside, when aired at all, with the bald statement that they gave consent.[61] But this is to ignore the broader question: why is women's reproductive labour not recognized as labour? It is because women's contribution to the production of stem cells is rarely recognized that the risks are little known. Because the risks are little known, and rarely publicized, the possibility of exploitation is obvious, both here and in commercial 'surrogacy'. There is an imbalance between the beneficiaries and the risk-takers in both therapeutic cloning and 'surrogacy'. Now imbalance is not in itself necessarily exploitative;[62] but when the risk-taking party is so invisible to the gaze of the beneficiaries as women are in the debates about these new reproductive technologies, the situation is ripe for exploitation. The very best way to exploit someone's labour is to pretend they're not working at all, and to get them to think so too – as Mark Twain noted in the tale of Tom Sawyer and the picket fence.

Why does no one notice women's labour? In philosophers from Aristotle to Marx, and in popular discourse too, what women do in giving life is like what the earth does: it is natural, not social, and it does not add surplus value. Now there is nothing natural about the new reproductive technologies, such as 'surrogacy' and therapeutic cloning, but we have not yet revised our image of what women do in providing the labour for these technologies, to view it as something other than natural, at best a 'labour of love'. As for adding surplus value, the value of stem cell lines can be expected to be enormous. We may or may not want women to reap those benefits: perhaps we might prefer a model that vests control in oocyte donors to a more limited extent – giving control over tissue to the mother, and treating un-authorized alienation of it from her as theft, as I have argued else-where.[63] But we certainly need to think harder about how to rectify the current risk–benefit equation, in which women bear all the physical risks but reap none of the benefits. Stem cell technologies highlight the 'use-value' which women produce in the reproductive labours of superovulation, egg extraction, and the work of early pregnancy and abortion. It is abundantly clear that these pregnancy-derived tissues have value, and enormous value.

What is shown by the commodification of bodily products such as stem cells is that there is no firm divide, as Marx thought there was, between the use-values produced through social means of production and the absence of use-values in reproduction. One effect of late capitalism – the commodification of practically everything – is to knock down the Chinese walls between the natural and productive realms, to use a Marxist framework.[64] Women's labour in egg extraction and 'surrogate' motherhood might then be seen for what it is, namely labour which produces something of value.[65] But this does not necessarily mean that women will benefit from the commodification of practically everything, in either North or South. In the newly developing biotechnologies involving stem cells, the reverse is more likely, particularly given the shortage in the North of the egg donors who will be increasingly necessary to therapeutic cloning. Instead of reaping the benefits of these technologies, women will disproportionately bear the risks – particularly women in the South, I think. Since the enucleated eggs needed in therapeutic cloning can be extracted from a woman of any race – after all, there is no nuclear content – I can foresee an aggravated, globalized disparity developing, where the benefits accrue to the wealthier citizens of the wealthier countries and the risks are borne by poor women in the developing countries.

Although most of the ethical debate has focused on the status of the embryo, this is to define ethics with no reference to global or gender justice. There has been little or no debate about possible exploitation of women, particularly of ovum donors from the South. Women in many sub-Saharan African countries, particularly, do not own their own reproductive labour.[66] Countries of the South without national ethics committees or guidelines may be particularly vulnerable: although there is increasing awareness of the susceptibility of poorer countries to abuses in *research* ethics, very little has been written about how they might be affected by the enormously profitable new technologies exploiting human tissue. Even in the UK, although the new Medical Research Council guidelines[67] make a good deal of the 'gift relationship', what they are actually about is commodification. If donors believe they are demonstrating altruism, but biotechnology firms and researchers use the discourse of commodity and profit, we have not 'incomplete commodification'[68] but complete commodification with a plausibly human face.

Vesting control over tissue in the mother may not be sufficient to protect the woman from exploitation by commercial interests. Those interests surpass any in 'surrogacy', where it is difficult enough to distinguish between allowing women to contract as equals and opening them to exploitation. Arguably, thinking of the mother as having any kind of property interest in foetal tissue or the tissue by-products of pregnancy is also false to the uniqueness of the relationship between the woman and the developing foetus.[69] Nevertheless, it is a start towards recognizing that women themselves should decide what risks they will bear.

Perhaps some might argue that researchers also take risks, albeit financial ones. Surplus value, they might say, is added not by the woman from whom the tissue is extracted, but by researchers and biotechnology firms. This was the argument accepted in the *Moore* judgement (1990), but it has also been argued that the *Moore* case was decided in a manner which breaches previous legal precedents.[70] The general principle in the common law (*res nullius*) has traditionally been that no one can hold property in tissue taken from the body. It may be that the patient does not own the tissue, but does that necessarily mean that the researcher or hospital does? If we wish to avoid the commodification of tissue that would result from allowing the patient tradeable rights, why are we so willing to allow them to the researchers? If we want to promote freedom of research, should we not restrict patents by biotechnology firms as much as we do the property rights of tissue-donating subjects? If we want to equalize the physical risks borne and the financial benefits accrued, should we not stop favouring researchers and biotechnology firms?

Normally, however, the discussion about women and stem cell tissue never even gets to the counter-argument stage. We simply do not notice that women are putting in labour through undergoing superovulation or egg extraction. Just as the women who actually take the risks of pregnancy and childbirth remain camouflaged under the term 'surrogate', the risks women bear in cloning technologies are simply not talked about. Because the risks to women are so little known, and because the few guidelines that do exist uniformly employ the 'language of gift', women cannot give a properly informed consent to the use of their oocytes in therapeutic cloning. Responsibility for ill-luck in outcomes cannot be transferred from researchers and clinicians to women who donate oocytes or labour in other ways in the new reproductive technologies, unless the risks are spelt out in advance. So the new reproductive technologies are consistent with the argument made about informed consent in chapter 4, but they take it one stage further. At least in the examples in chapter 4 we knew who the patient was, and we knew that her consent was required. In cloning, women as the real patients or research subjects have been invisible: only the clone and the embryo are considered to be visible and vulnerable.

8

Psychiatry and Risk

This chapter will explore the risk assessments made by practitioners considering whether to release mentally disordered patients who may be a danger to themselves or to others. In these cases 'getting it wrong' makes a great deal of difference, but is the clinician morally responsible if the outcome judged less probable does in fact occur? How can clinicians balance uncertainty and risk with their duty of care? Three anonymized cases drawn from clinical practice will be examined in the first part of the chapter – the first two more dramatic, concerning primarily risk of harm to others, and the third more 'everyday', concerning risk of harm to self. All these issues deal primarily with luck in outcomes, which is the subject of the first part of this chapter; but there is also another sort of moral luck to which psychiatry is particularly relevant, luck in character. The case that will be examined in the second part of the chapter, however, transcends ill-luck in character. It concerns ill-luck in the very possibility of having a moral character in the first place.

Risk and dangerousness: luck in outcomes

What would it take to 'get it right' in making judgements of dangerousness and risk? There are two difficulties about 'getting it right'. One is the question, rehearsed elsewhere in this book and particularly in chapter 4 on informed consent, of whether the question is getting the outcome right or getting the procedure right. I argued strongly for the latter in chapter 4 and do not intend to repeat that argument here. The second difficulty has not been fully dealt with. It concerns the element of utility as well as probability in clinical assessments of risk.

In the risk assessment literature 'dangerousness' is often distinguished from risk as being the more value-laden concept.[1] What counts as dangerous to one person, in one context, may not seem dangerous to another. There are obvious gender questions here, among others. But is the concept of 'risk' itself value-free? Not insofar as risk is composed of both probability and utility. To non-Bayesians, at least, probability appears objective and value-free, but utility is specifically subjective: it is the value that individual agents attach to particular outcomes. In the following real but heavily anonymized case[2] the tension is created in part by the differing utilities that different providers of psychiatric services attach to different outcomes – depending on whether those outcomes concern the patient or his children. Merely agreeing on the risk of the patient's dangerousness to himself and his children would not therefore have resolved the disagreement.

Alan Masterson, aged fifty-four, was referred to psychiatric services for depression the year after he lost his management job in a corporate 'restructuring'. His general practitioner was concerned about his serious weight loss, which had no physiological cause. Alan reported fleeting suicidal wishes, along with sleeplessness and marital tension. Although he felt guilty about having lost his job, he thought that was not the only factor in his mental state. Depression seemed to 'run in the family', he said; his mother had also suffered from it and had become more or less of a recluse in her later years, refusing even to see her grandchildren. He described himself likewise as 'a bit of a loner, not a team player': 'I suppose I was never really cut out for management, it's a wonder I lasted as long as I did.' Luckily there was no immediate financial pressure: Alan had received a sizeable redundancy payment from his well-paid position, and his wife Valerie worked as an architect's receptionist. Nevertheless he was very pessimistic about the financial future, repeatedly predicting that his wife and sons would end up in a council house and he would wind up in a cardboard box at Waterloo station. The senior registrar working with Alan, Anya Washansky, decided that he should be maintained on antidepressants, with a referral to marriage guidance and follow-up in the outpatients department.

Six months later, however, Alan was admitted to a psychiatric ward after his three sons were very nearly electrocuted. The children were swimming in the family pool, and the eldest, thirteen-year-old Tom, had left a portable CD player plugged in to recharge on a long lead attached to the electrical point in the machinery which housed the pool heater. As Tom told the story, his father deliberately threw the CD player into the pool; as Alan told it, he tripped over the wire and the player catapulted into the water. By great good fortune the CD player, which had only been loosely plugged in, flew out of the electrical point just before it fell into the water. No one else saw the incident; the two younger boys were roughhousing together with their backs to their father, and Alan's wife Valerie was out at work. She believed Tom's version of events, and was of course greatly distraught – and very angry with Anya for failing to protect the boys from Alan. She had immediately phoned the police, and child protection machinery was set in motion, including referral to Social Services.

Alan denied to Anya that he had tried to kill the boys, although he did say that his sons would be 'better off dead than stuck with a loser like me for a dad'. However, he did agree to emergency admission on an informal basis, admitting that he had not been taking his antidepressants: 'I can't be bothered, maybe it's better if you make me do it.' In the ward Alan was given a further trial of a tricyclic antidepressant, but without much apparent benefit: he still had depressed mood and suicidal thoughts. He continued to deny that he had tried to kill the boys: 'Kids have accidents all the time, don't they?'

During Alan's period in hospital Social Services and the police both requested further information from the mental health team. The police requested a psychiatric opinion on Alan's fitness to be interviewed, in the presence of a psychiatric nurse. Their opinion was that it was unlikely that Alan would be prosecuted; at most a formal caution might be given, but more likely there would be insufficient evidence to prosecute. However, they requested a forensic opinion on the risk posed to the children. This latter request the mental health team was willing to grant, although they did not consider Alan was yet ready to be interviewed by the police.

In contrast, the Social Services request for more detail on the swimming pool incident and on Alan's previous treatment in outpatients met with a refusal from the psychiatrists, on grounds of patient confidentiality. Nor would they reveal Alan's discharge date to Social Services. On the advice of her consultant, Paul Glover, Anya informed Social Services that it was the responsibility of Alan's wife Valerie to do so, when Alan returned home. Paul felt that it was the mental health team's duty to put Alan's medical needs first, whereas Social Services's primary responsibility was to protect the children. While Paul realized the possible risks to the boys, he felt that their future lay in making Alan well again. And his primary duty was to respect the therapeutic relationship, which would be shattered if Alan felt that the psychiatrists were not fully on 'his' side, and if information which he had revealed in confidence was divulged. Alan was not the easiest person to engage in conversation: he was often morose and taciturn. And after all, Alan had been admitted informally, so that he could discharge himself at any time: surely the best long-term protection for the boys, too, lay in maintaining an atmosphere in which Alan voluntarily accepted help. In his letter to Social Services, Paul took what he thought was a concili-atory tone, agreeing that Alan was 'certainly a risk to himself'. He assured them that treatments were in hand, although he did not specif-ically mention that Alan was due to have an MRI scan soon and a course of electroplexy if the scan proved to be normal.

This response occasioned a swift written protest from the Social Services Department, sent in the first instance to Paul, but with copies to senior social services, hospital trust and health authority manage-ment. The service manager, Kathy McAllister, viewed this as a totally improper interpretation of patient confidentiality, and as unreasonable withholding of information necessary for Social Services to carry out its statutory child protection responsibilities. Social Services had decided to defer putting the children on the At Risk Register so long as Alan was in hospital and the children therefore safe. But there was still an urgent need for full exchange of information. And why was the mental health team only concerned that Alan was a risk to *himself*, when vulnerable children were in danger?

For understandable reasons, mental health and social services are likely to have different attitudes towards risk assessment and risk aversion. To a large extent, this incompatibility results from having different objects of concern, of being responsible in the one case for the adult patient and in the other for the vulnerable child. The question of 'protecting whom', of the proper object of one's profes-sional duty, will be explored further in a moment. But different atti-tudes towards risk assessment are not explained solely by different objects of responsibility. There is also the important question of how things can go wrong, and how they can go wrong in different ways for the two sets of professionals. This is where the issue of luck in outcomes comes in.

What counts as 'getting it wrong' in psychiatry? To the extent that a medical model obtains,[3] the answer is 'failing to cure'. It is the possibility of cure that underpins the therapeutic relationship in psychiatry, although, as in all areas of medicine – avowedly so in palliative care – the alleviation of suffering might more properly be construed as the goal. However, most clinicians admit that there are some boundaries on the sanctity of the therapeutic relationship, such as patient autonomy or public protection. It is in the name of protect-ing the public that the General Medical Council guidelines clearly state that there are limits to patient confidentiality, such as the actual duty to report suspected child abuse.[4] (Clearly a non-consequentialist view is visible here: the positive outcome, cure, does not justify trespass against certain duties, or certain virtues, in the medical professional.) Perhaps the clinicians are more concerned with social harm – the possibility that Alan will never see his children again if he is deemed a risk to them. For whatever reason, it does appear that Alan's clinicians are concerned with preserving the therapeutic relationship from outside 'intrusion', and with avoiding the breakdown of the therapeutic relationship that they feel a breach of confidentiality may provoke. Although they are of course concerned with the boys' welfare too, they may think they have reason to feel that it is by no means certain that Alan tried to kill his sons.

For social services child protection staff, however, 'getting it wrong' means failing to protect vulnerable children. The extreme of 'getting it wrong' would be the boys' deaths. Because that harm is so very great – in itself, not only because it would almost certainly lead to media denunciations – social services are unwilling to tolerate even a very small probability of its occurrence. This is a perfectly rational attitude, exemplifying the logic in Pascal's Wager:[5] a loss which approaches infinity in its magnitude is so great as to cancel out all probability considerations. No matter how unlikely the harm may be, even the smallest probability of it is intolerable. It is not so much a matter of necessarily believing Tom's account of the swimming pool incident over Alan's, as of fearing the consequences of not preferring Tom's account more.

Must we simply accept that the two services have differing attitudes towards risk assessment, and ne'er the twain shall meet? To the extent that the law favours one interpretation over the other, that view of risk assessment must be accepted. As Kathy McAllister points out, social services child protection staff must be given sufficient information to fulfil their statutory obligations. However, that does not necessarily entail full information-sharing, as she claims: there may be some room for compromise over what information social services genuinely need to know. But there is a significant risk here. *Withholding information means that one bears full responsibility for an adverse outcome*, where sharing information with patients or other agencies might have averted tragedy. There is a parallel here with my argument about consent in chapter 4: it is against doctors' own interest in avoiding remorse to be the sole 'owners' of crucial information.

There is also a question about to whom the professional's duty is owed, and that, too, will affect the utility calculation. Some people's interests may count more in the risk equation than others'. Might Paul and Anya be said to have a duty to Alan's children as well? Could that duty be even more pressing than their duty to protect Alan's best interests – perhaps because children are more vulnerable than adult patients? That seems an unpromising line of argument, however: particular children might be less vulnerable than extremely ill psychiatric patients. The extent of duty cannot hinge on ready-reckoning the extent of vulnerability. For one thing, there would be moral luck problems in doing so: if things did indeed go dreadfully wrong, we might not know the extent of vulnerability until later.

In a contractual interpretation of medicine, the doctor–patient relationship would be primary because a sort of contract had been put into effect between those two parties when the patient sought care. The duties specified by such a contract might include complying with treatment and providing necessary information on the part of the patient, provision of best available service and honouring of patients' reasonable wishes on the part of the doctor. But although contractual models are increasingly influential in public policy,[6] they are not the legal basis of health care, at least not in the National Health Service, where there is no actual contract between patient and doctor.

Contract is a useful metaphor in ethics – whatever its merits or demerits in law – for recognizing others as active agents rather than as passive objects of concern, and indeed I have argued elsewhere for such a Hegelian approach to contract.[7] But in this case there does not seem to be a great deal of mileage in a contractual approach. It will not bridge the abyss between mental health and social services, only widen it, if the psychiatrists insist that their 'contract' is with Alan and Alan alone, regardless of the danger to his children, who are the statutory responsibility of the social services. And Alan's wife Valerie will be left out of the equation altogether. We might not want to go so far as to say that the clinicians have a duty to her, but she feels badly let down by them.

If the clinician's duties are construed too extensively, however, we encounter what Thomas Nagel terms 'the problem of excess objectivity'. It is important to amplify our concern, beyond the doctor–patient dyad, to take the wider world into account, and this the contractual model fails to do. Yet the opposite risk is to make the clinician responsible for too much, and, ironically, to erase her sense of moral efficacy. Once we expand beyond the doctor–patient relationship, and include the wider world in calculations of moral duty, we may be so overwhelmed by everything we are obliged to take into account that we can see no point in acting at all.

> Once people are seen as being parts of the world, there seems no way to assign responsibility to them for what they do. Everything about them, including finally their actions themselves, seems to blend in with the surroundings over which they have no control.[8]

This is the problem of excess objectivity. Nagel's nearest thing to a solution is 'a kind of reconciliation between the objective standpoint and the inner perspective of agency which reduces the radical detachment produced by initial contemplation of ourselves as creatures in the world.' Specifically in relation to the problem of moral luck and responsibility, he suggests the maxim that we have already encountered: 'Since we can't act in light of everything about ourselves, the best we can do is to try to live in a way that wouldn't have to be revised in light of anything more that could be known about us.'[9]

How can this be applied to Alan's case? Anya and Paul cannot act in light of everything that could be known about Alan's future risk to his sons, but they can try to live in such a way that they will not regret their actions if the unexpected occurs. It appears that the unexpected, to them, would be for Tom's version of events to have been the correct one: for Alan to discharge himself prematurely, with no improvement, for social services to be unable to act because they have not been told the discharge date and Valerie does not notify them, and for the boys to die in an 'accident' of Alan's contriving. If that worst case occurred, Anya and Paul might not be directly responsible for the boys' deaths, but they would be responsible for a certain kind of professional arrogance in thinking they could ignore the worst-case scenario.

Another anonymized real-life case also raises issues concerning ill-luck in outcomes. Although the immediate issue in the Alan Masterson case is confidentiality, rather than consent to treatment,[10] one might argue that the underlying question in both consent and confidentiality is who should bear responsibility for ill-luck in outcomes if the clinician keeps all the information to herself. The case of Alan Masterson thus indirectly reinforced my argument that giving information and getting consent obviates the clinician's responsibility if things go wrong. The second case in this section puts the issue of consent more directly in the foreground and also draws our attention to the several ways in which things can go wrong.

Philip Caversham, now in his early forties, was cautioned for an indecent exposure involving a schoolgirl when he was twenty-eight. Since then he has served a period of probation and a prison sentence, both for indecent assault. He has had lifelong psychosexual problems: his marriage was never consummated, and his wife divorced him after his prison sentence. The first psychiatric assessment only took place some years after he had begun to offend, while he was in prison. He was diagnosed as suffering from paranoid schizophrenia and was treated with injected antipsychotic drugs. However, he does not accept this diagnosis; instead he claims that his ordeal in prison accounts for his psychiatric problems. His sense of grievance against the psychiatric profession is considerable, and he categorically denies that there is anything wrong with him.

Since his release two years ago Philip has committed no further offences and has had no hospital admissions. He used to attend a psychiatric outpatient clinic erratically, but accepted merely the very minimum level of medication by injection, claiming that the drugs were poisonous. It seems that he only attended the clinic because he dreaded being 'sectioned' or imprisoned again. His behaviour in the clinic was always very eccentric: he stared around the room while talking, casting the occasional darting glance at the interviewer before looking hurriedly away in a manner suggesting delusions of thought interference – although he rejected any such interpretation with outrage. He would terminate any attempt at interview abruptly, usually with cutting remarks about the skills and training of his clinicians, Nick Fox and Margaret Shanley. Nick and Margaret felt that only an increased dosage would protect him in the long term from psychotic relapse, but Philip was very hostile to any such suggestions. He refused to participate in any care planning or assessment.

About ten months ago, when interviewed in the presence of Parvadi Mehta, a second-year clinical medical student, Philip became extremely agitated. He stared at her pointedly, shouting that the girls he assaulted had 'asked for it'. This was the first time he had spoken of his offences; in the past he always refused to discuss them. A month later, in an interview designed to assess his risk of further sexual offending, he spoke out angrily in a similar vein about 'slags'. After that Philip disappeared from follow-up altogether, but sent a coherent letter, claiming that he had been misunderstood in both interviews. He was willing to return for follow-up only on condition that there was no further insulting talk of delusions or psychosis. Nor was he willing to accept any more drugs, he stipulated. Anyone the 'shrinks' think well enough to live in 'the so-called community', he remarked tartly, was well enough to refuse drugs. His sexuality had been channelled into art, he claimed; recently he gave an exhibition of his amateur paintings –

proof, he said, that he was flourishing without the psychiatrists' interference. But whereas he told the clinical team that he painted land-
scapes, they know that he is actually primarily interested in female
nudes.

The clinicians' preferred management would be to increase Philip's
medication, see him more often, refer him to a forensic psychiatrist to
get a risk estimate for re-offending, and finally, place him on the
hospital supervision register. They are concerned about the two violent
outbursts, and fear that Philip's condition is declining rather than
improving, as he insists it is. But if they call him in to discuss these
courses of action, Philip is likely to break off even the minimal contact
he now has. Placing him on the supervision register, unlike the other
three courses, could be done without his knowledge or co-operation.
But given that there are no new resources available, what would it
achieve? Perhaps it would only stigmatize Philip without offering him
any extra help.

Nick and Margaret have considered whether it might improve Philip's
compliance with long-term management to keep the supervision register
in reserve as a threat, along the lines of 'sectioning' – which he does seem
to respect. This they find preferable to the harder approach that they
could actually take under aftercare legislation – conveying Philip to a
treatment centre without his consent. On the other hand, if Philip were
to find out that he had been placed on the supervision register behind his
back, it might only increase his hostility to the doctors. Ironically, by
placing him on the supervision register, Nick and Margaret feel that they
would lose the last shreds of their ability to supervise him.

Philip and his clinicians, Nick and Margaret, are at odds over the
correct interpretation of his behaviour, and thereby over his future
dangerousness. Whose version should prevail? It is the risk of harm to
others that gives the clinicians' version greater potential legitimacy.
They cannot just take Philip at his word, given his history of
offending. Equally, however, they cannot be certain that he will offend
again, and indeed he offers a coherent if not entirely plausible argument about why he is unlikely to do so. So the problem boils down to
assessing the risk, which in turn dictates what treatment, if any,
should be imposed, with or without Philip's consent.

How much intervention can be justified by future risk of harm to
others? An initial means of gaining some purchase on the question of
risk assessment in Philip's case might seem to be the notion of significant harm in child protection legislation – in England and Wales, for
example, in the Children Act 1989. Evidence that harm has occurred
in the past is not enough, unless it points to significant likelihood of

harm continuing into the future.[11] Do Philip's actions point, then, to significant likelihood of future harm? His self-justification in terms of channelling his sexuality into art sounds rather specious, and there may well be danger to the models he paints or to the schoolgirls he passes in the street. But because these risks are only probabilities for a statistical aggregate, we cannot yet say for certain that any particular girl or woman is in danger. Here the parallel with child protection breaks down: typically the child on the 'at risk' register is at risk from known adults.

The example of Philip Caversham is a case about risk assessment in building up a diagnosis and treatment plan, and about what might happen if that process of evaluation goes wrong. That is, if things turn out badly, who bears the responsibility? If no further treatment is imposed on Philip except his self-imposed art 'therapy', he may well reoffend – and then what? In the United States, practitioners have still been found civilly liable for releasing patients who have since harmed others.[12]

The concepts 'moral' or 'ethical' feel incompatible with that of 'luck' for clinicians, who are likely to be blamed for irresponsible or unprofessional behaviour if they get treatment decisions wrong – and, even more importantly, to blame themselves too. If Nick and Margaret decide not to exercise their powers to place Philip on the supervision register or to convey him to a treatment centre, and another girl is assaulted, will they reproach themselves? There seems to be something deeply wrong with the prospect of the clinicians shrugging such an assault off as just bad luck. Yet, in another sense, what Philip decides to do is beyond their control: he would be the agent who commits the crime. And long-term management in the community gives the practitioner less control over the patient, compared with the ward situation.

Is the psychiatrist who decides not to take out a supervision order or to place a possibly dangerous person on a supervision register morally at fault if that person harms someone, or merely unlucky? What would be the appropriate reaction for the clinician who 'gets it wrong?' The examples of Philip Caversham and Alan Masterson extend the meaning of 'getting it wrong' – not only for the patient, but also for family members or the public at large. In the section on remorse and regret in chapter 3, I argued that the language of preference-maximization was alien to medicine because of the doctor's duty of care to the patient. If there is also some sort of duty to others than the patient, the 'ante' is 'upped' even further. There seems to be no limit to the remorse a conscientious professional might feel if things go wrong not just for the patient, but also for others at risk of serious harm, even death, as a result of the patient's actions.

It is too much to ask that Nick and Margaret should feel that they have failed personally if Philip commits another assault. Remorse, or Williams's near-substitute, agent-regret, seems a certain route to guilt, burnout and disillusionment among the most conscientious clinicians. It also implies a kind of *hubris* or fatal arrogance: only an all-seeing divine judge could know everything that bears on a decision and always give the right weight to it. Yet Williams is right to dismiss as 'very importantly wrong' the view that we can always avoid self-criticism if we have considered all available information carefully before making the decision and have done everything possible to avoid the unfortunate outcome.[13] Such a perspective involves an unhealthy distance from one's own actions, and a failure to distinguish ethical dilemmas from ordinary practical rationality – prudential decisions, such as which car to buy.

Let us return to what moral luck implies about risk and consent in cases such as Philip's, where the clinicians' assessment differs from that of the patient. A focus on ill-luck in outcomes concentrates the mind wonderfully: although the most obvious way in which things could turn out badly would be for Philip to reoffend, there are actually two ways in which things could turn out badly in this particular case. Philip's therapeutic outcome could be worsened, the clinicians feel, if they place him on the supervision register without his consent.

The only way in which the conscientious clinician can avoid remorse if things go badly wrong for the patient or for others harmed by the patient is to respect the *a priori* principle of obtaining informed consent. (This is, of course, a Kantian rather than a utilitarian argument, consistent with the discussion in chapters 2 and 3.) If Nick and Margaret bypass the consent procedures, then they bear the responsibility for any worsening in Philip's condition, against their expectations of therapeutic success. This may appear to put the clinicians in a cleft stick: damned if they seek Philip's consent to being put on the supervision register and he absconds altogether, damned if they don't and he finds out they have acted behind his back, destroying what little therapeutic alliance has been constructed. Of the two possible adverse outcomes – and it is important to recognize that both *are* possible – the second should actually occasion more self-blame in the clinicians than the first. The first is Philip's choice, not Nick and Margaret's.

In neither of the first two case studies did withholding information seem justified. The third case is more problematic, because the patient is clearly not capable of understanding the information and giving consent.

Gilbert Ryan, a 79-year-old widower, lives with his learning-disabled son Stephen in sheltered housing. He has mild to moderate Alzheimer's Disease, with very poor short-term memory. His language abilities are reasonably well preserved, as is his mobility. Always very active as a younger man, Gilbert still enjoys 'getting out and about', as he puts it. 'Got to get some air.'

The difficulty is that now his 'getting out and about' has got out of control. Up until now the problems were confined to Gilbert's uncertainty over which of the sheltered housing flats was his own, when he came back from walks with his dog Barney. This was not too serious: Stephen, who is very attached to Gilbert, was usually waiting at the gate to fetch his father back home. But now Gilbert has taken to wandering in the very early hours of the morning, when Stephen is still asleep. Gilbert normally wakes around three a.m., but sometimes rises several times during the night, at unpredictable hours.

Several times Gilbert was found by the milkman, near the entrance to the flats. But two months ago, in January, things took a sudden turn for the worse. After going missing for an entire day Gilbert was located unconscious, a mile away, in a ditch with the dog: the victim of a hit-and-run motorist. Luckily Barney's body heat was detected by the search team, using a heat detector. Gilbert's own body temperature had fallen so low as to be undetectable.

Fortunately there were no serious injuries. Gilbert recovered in hospital and was then admitted informally as an emergency case to a psychogeriatric unit. His sleep patterns have become more settled with mild night-time sedation, and a urinary infection, which might have caused his restlessness, is now under control. At first he desperately wanted to return home to Stephen, but after ten days, he is now less keen to leave the ward. However, he does not want his mobility impaired by sedative drugs: getting out and about is still his major preoccupation.

Gilbert's consultant, Hassan Shah, has called a case conference to discuss the risk management issues. Gilbert is very hesitant when crossing the road, in observations of his traffic assessment. When he does start to cross, he is unable to react to drivers. Hassan is not at all happy about releasing Gilbert to return home. But if the risks of a trial at home are considered acceptable by the case conference, he would like to stipulate that a tracking device should be part of the care package. He has tried to talk about tracking to Gilbert during his intervals of competence, but has not succeeded in getting a meaningful consent. Whether this is due to Gilbert's inability to remember and understand the options, or to outright opposition, seems unclear. Stephen does not understand the idea of tracking, but he is enthusiastic about it because then he can have 'Dad home'.

Jane Vargos, a senior social worker who is 'Approved' under the Mental Health Act to deal with compulsory admission of at-risk patients, warns that Social Services policy on tracking is very stringent. She might be subject to disciplinary action if she approved it. An additional difficulty is that Social Services do not have any money to fund placement of patients in nursing homes, except on a strictly one-to-one basis. This means that in-patient psychogeriatric units, often needed as part of the emergency management of patients who wander, will be increasingly less able to respond to such emergencies, because their beds will be blocked by patients awaiting placement in nursing homes. The implications are that patients with wandering problems will increasingly be managed in the community, with the increased exposure to risk that this necessarily entails.

On the face of it, then, fitting Gilbert with a tracking device preserves the frequently cited, if rather formulaic, principles of autonomy, beneficence and non-maleficence (first do no harm). But what if the device isn't foolproof? Suppose a failure of the device leaves Gilbert lying in a ditch again, when he could be safe in hospital. Wouldn't the clinicians be responsible – if they relied too heavily on tracking as a substitute for proper supervision? That raises not only pragmatic issues, but also issues about moral luck.

Normally, as I have argued before in this book, it is the giving of informed consent to treatment that transfers responsibility for ill-luck in outcomes from doctor to patient, within the limits of negligence. Although a tracking device is not treatment as such, it is part of the treatment or management plan for Gilbert, so that issues of consent do arise. If Gilbert does not give a consent that Hassan Shah regards as satisfactory, is it impermissible to fit him with a tracking device? Contrariwise, if he does consent, can he be said to have taken responsibility for any future ill-luck in outcomes – including the worst-case scenario in which the device malfunctions, leaving him dead in the ditch?

Here the risk is to Gilbert himself, rather than to others, as in the previous two cases. Although Gilbert's mental capacity to give an informed consent is not fully established, even a person whose competence is not in doubt is not permitted to take any and all risks – not if their risk-taking poses unnecessary intolerable harm to others. This is what motorway speed limits are about. The difference here is that Gilbert poses a risk primarily to himself: he is the one likely to be knocked over, perhaps killed this time, if his wandering is not monitored. But the right to risk self-harm is rarely unqualified – because other people usually get hurt too, although perhaps in less obvious ways. In this case, Stephen will be shattered if anything happens to his father. More broadly, 'the wandering old man who gets knocked down in the road has inflicted harm on the driver as well as himself.'[14] Even the hit-and-run driver may have had a conscience, which must now be troubled.

There is at present, in contrast to many American jurisdictions,[15] no doctrine of proxy or substituted consent in English law, not even for adults lacking mental capacity. (This position may change in England and Wales if proposals put forward by the Law Commission and the Department of Health are enacted into statute.[16] In Scotland a similar statute involving adults with mental incapacity was passed in 2000.) This means that no one else, not even a family member, can give consent on Gilbert's behalf – not Stephen, for example, even if he were capable of fully understanding what tracking involves. It also means that no one else, apart from the clinician, can shoulder the blame if things go wrong. If the patient's informed consent has not been obtained, then risk cannot be said to be transferred from clinician to patient. This appears to be a stumbling-block for my earlier position: that consent functions to transfer responsibility for ill-luck in outcomes. If no one can give a valid consent, then who bears the responsibility if things go wrong?

It is difficult to see how we can escape from this dilemma without recourse to the doctrine of best interests. If an adult patient lacks mental capacity, no one else can consent on his or her behalf. In this case the general principle in English law is that the doctor is justified in acting in the name of the patient's best interests. The problem highlighted by moral luck is that that judgement of what is in the patient's best interests may be 'flawed' in one of three ways. It may be coloured by the doctor's own values or utilities, as, for example, when doctors assume that treatment is always preferable to no treatment. Or it may be based on an inaccurate assessment of probabilities. However, the third possibility also remains: when the doctor's judgement of the patient's best interests is reasonably dispassionate in utility terms, and well-calibrated in probability terms, but results in an unfavourable outcome nevertheless. It is the third case that is troubling where a valid informed consent cannot be obtained, as will frequently be the case in psychiatry. This is not true because people with mental illness necessarily lack mental capacity; the law retains the presumption of competence in the case of adult patients with mental illness.[17] The problem is that there is no one else to assume responsibility for ill-luck in outcomes, through a valid informed consent, in the case of an adult patient whose competence is in doubt. Some, though by no means all, adult patients with mental illness will fall into that category.

I argued in chapter 4 that it was the giving of genuine informed consent that stopped the probability machine rolling, and that absolved the doctor from feeling remorse, although regret might remain. Perhaps one thing we might say is that, where an adult patient cannot give an informed consent, where the psychiatrist makes a decision based on the patient's best interests, and where that decision turns out badly, the psychiatrist should still be expected to feel nothing more than regret. Remorse is not an option, in a way. How helpful this is to practising clinicians is another matter. If the clinical team decide to fit Gilbert with a tracking device 'in his best interests' and to relax their supervision, and if he then winds up dead in a ditch, having ripped the device off, they may well feel remorseful, even if Gilbert himself is partially implicated, and even if Gilbert could not give a valid consent.

Perhaps they are likely to feel remorse *because* they are patient-centred clinicians, unlike, say, the radiographer in chapter 4. Recall the latter's reaction to the death of one of his patients, who had not been told of a serious risk:

> I have done 6000 to 8000 urograms in the past thirteen years and no one has ever had a fatal reaction. We have been doing urograms at this hospital for at least 25 years, and no one has ever had a fatal reaction... Because the indications for urography were great and the chances for a reaction were remote, I am sure I would have convinced Mrs E ... to have the procedures. She would have then had the reaction and died, and the fact that I warned her would have done Mrs E ... absolutely no good.[18]

The urographer, although dealing with a patient whose mental capacity was not in doubt, gives his paternalism away with his talk of 'convincing' Mrs E. The clinicians in Gilbert's case, dealing with a patient whose competence is seriously in doubt, seem to be doing their best to enhance Gilbert's competence – not least by allowing him to 'get up and about' rather than become housebound or institutionalized. He is already less keen to leave the ward: the risks to be considered must include the undesirable outcome of institutionalized behaviour too.

In chapter 4 I argued for an absolutist approach to consent. This chapter's psychiatry-centred discussion suggests that I was in fact somewhat too absolutist. Where informed consent cannot be obtained from the adult patient who lacks capacity, we are forced to revert to the usually paternalistic 'best interests' standard. No one else can assume responsibility for ill-luck in outcomes: family members cannot give or withhold consent on behalf of an incompetent adult patient. Nor, in a case like Gilbert's, can the patient himself fully assume that responsibility.

We are left with a heavy burden of responsibility if things go wrong, and with no one's shoulders available to carry it but the clinician's. It does not seem just to impose that on the doctor who genuinely tries to maximize patients' ability to give consent, and who follows best practice and legal guidelines about consent as functional to this specific decision rather than as all-embracing. Even with changes towards a more flexible standard of mental capacity, there will still be patients who cannot give consent. The most we can say is that the doctor who genuinely tries to transfer that responsibility for ill-luck in outcomes through obtaining the patient's informed consent, but who cannot do so, should not be held accountable if things turn out wrong. Her project may have failed, but she has not failed, in Williams's terms. Remorse is not appropriate, although regret may be.

Luck in character

In the three cases above, I focused primarily on luck in outcomes, but luck in character may also be relevant, particularly to the first two. (Gilbert's case is more about cognitive inability rather than anything like character deficiency.) A virtue-ethics approach would want to say something about Philip's and Alan's characters, not just about the consequences of their actions. I think a Kantian approach would too, insofar as neither man is making himself an autonomous member of the kingdom of ends: both are driven by their depression or psychoses. The question of responsibility, however, is common to both parts of this chapter.

As Claudia Card reminds us in her analysis of moral luck and character, our characters are shaped by what we are held responsible for.[19] The paradox of moral luck concerns the simultaneous requirements that we should be held responsible only for what we can control, and that we should realize people often cannot control very much. What does seem within our control is the 'good will', in Kantian terms, even if external outcomes are beyond our shaping. Psychiatry, however, offers many examples of people whose will seems to be determined largely by external events, particularly those in the grip of psychoses. It has been argued that psychosis consists precisely in the absence of a sense of moral agency, not in the content of delusions, and that it should therefore be understood as much in moral as in clinical terms.[20] There are real problems about whether moral agency is compatible with that view of a person, and about whether the Kantian emphasis on the good will can withstand the example of the person who has no will at all, good or otherwise. Even if we cannot control external events, we should be able to control our response to them, to generate an identity as autonomous agents, to bring our characters or wills under our own agency.

In some extreme cases, the most severe kind of ill-luck in character would conceivably be to have no such thing as a character. The following case study illustrates the difficulty of holding the patient responsible for very much at all.

Delia Jarrett is a 35-year-old woman with an extensive psychiatric history, dating back to the age of sixteen. Diagnoses of her condition have been many and various, including personality disorder, substance abuse, bipolar affective disorder, schizo-affective disorder, schizophrenia, and various combinations of the above.

She and her older brother Thomas were raised by an elderly aunt and uncle in Barbados, after their parents' deaths in a traffic accident during Delia's early childhood. When Delia was twelve the family emigrated to Britain, and she attended a local comprehensive school, where her behaviour was normal for some time. At fifteen, however, she began to play truant, to shoplift, and to abuse drugs. The next year she gave birth to a full-term baby, which was subsequently adopted.

Her first contact with psychiatric services came shortly afterwards, when she was found wandering down an airport runway while a plane was trying to land. She told the airport authorities that she was chasing the pretty lights of the plane, but informed police that she was trying to get a lift to see some friends. Delia was admitted informally but then detained under a section of the Mental Health Act. During her stay, which lasted approximately one month, she was diagnosed as manic and treated with Haloperidol, up to 90 mg per day. As on many subsequent admissions, however, the issue of drug abuse just prior to contact with psychiatric services could not be ruled out, although she claimed not to be using drugs at the time. Following discharge, which was rapid and unplanned, she quickly dropped out of contact with psychiatric services, despite clinicians' efforts to stay in touch.

By the time Delia was eighteen, her aunt and uncle had died, and she came into a small inheritance from them, which she spent on a holiday in Africa for herself and a boyfriend. During the holiday she was admitted on a compulsory basis to a psychiatric hospital, and her boyfriend abandoned her. Her brother Thomas had to fly out and bring her back home. This became a pattern: throughout her life Delia has repeatedly returned to Thomas for help, promising not to lead such a disorganized life. Her brother has complained to psychiatric services that Delia is completely irresponsible: she cannot feed or clothe herself reliably, cannot manage money, is often aggressive and sometimes violent, abuses drugs, and once tried to set fire to his house. Although Thomas has helped her financially many times, he has now taken out an interdict against her coming back to his home. But she has taken to breaking in and causing damage when her brother and his wife are not there.

Delia's subsequent admissions have often followed incidents in which she has been picked up by police. In one case, she stole a car but was placed on probation for a year after the responsible psychiatrist stated that her mental state would have affected her actions and her capacity to form the intention to commit a crime. In another instance, she was arrested after wandering around in the middle of the city streets, jumping in front of passing cars. On admission her thought was disordered, and she appeared to be visually hallucinated. She insisted that she had killed a baby, and also that she was pregnant. Her urine showed the presence of amphetamines. Again she was detained under a section of the Mental Health Act, remaining in hospital for ten weeks with a diagnosis of hypomania and probable personality disorder. She required high doses of neuroleptics, which seem to control acute episodes of mental illness but to have little effect on her behavioural problems. And again there was doubt as to whether she was really mentally ill, had a personality disorder, was abusing illicit substances – or possibly a combination of all three.

Discharged to a therapeutic community, Delia deliberately sabotaged her placement, as she admitted later, by smearing faeces and splashing urine in the toilet. She then dropped out of regular contact with psychiatric services and returned to a drug-dealing boyfriend, who was known to be violent to her. A complaint was made by the local branch of MIND about gross inadequacies in provision of care, accusing the hospital of turning a blind eye. Delia was now wandering the streets barefoot, talking to imaginary companions, and wandering in and out of traffic. The consultant concerned, Samantha George, replied that compulsory admissions and drug therapies had shown no long-term improvements in Delia's condition. She added that she was not sure that Delia had ever been mentally ill, and that she wondered if past admissions had been due to intoxication or other drug abuse. Meanwhile, Delia has just been arrested again – after throwing a brick through the window of a police car that was standing at traffic lights, barely missing the driver. She told the locum senior registrar that she was hearing voices telling her to go to prison. When asked whether she realised that she could have killed somebody, she replied, 'As long as it's a policeman, that's all right.'

There is considerable doubt among the clinical team about whether Delia has ever been frankly psychotic, but her reasoning is often so bizarre that mental disorder must be suspected. Although medication seems to help in the short term, it does result in severe side effects, worsening her restlessness. The clinicians have persisted pragmatically with a low-dose depot regime, but she often defaults from her appointments. To complicate the picture yet further, her behaviour does seem to improve while she is in hospital if staff impose strict guidelines, stating clearly what is acceptable and unacceptable. It is unclear therefore how much of her behaviour is under her own control.

There are two general conditions, very roughly speaking, which must be fulfilled before attributing responsibility for an action:[21] (1) the agent knows what she is doing; (2) the agent's desires and /or intentions influence the action. Are these conditions met in Delia's case? We might have considerable doubts about condition (1). On the one hand, Delia's behaviour does improve if staff set strict guidelines. This seems to indicate that she knows both what she is doing and that it is unacceptable. Conversely, depot medication does not improve her behaviour greatly once she is out of the controlled hospital environment in which staff can set guidelines for her. So, again, her behaviour seems to be under her conscious control, and not simply determined by psychopharmacology.

But what would it mean to say that Delia freely chooses how she acts? Isn't this much too hard on her? There is a strong element of disabling compulsion in her behaviour, the opposite of free choice. This view – meaning that she is *not* really responsible for her actions – predominated in the testimony of the psychiatrist at Delia's trial for car theft. Her mental state, in his opinion, affected her capacity to form an intention, in this case a criminal intention.

However, even a diagnosis of mental illness does not itself establish – in either ethics or law – that a person is definitely *not* responsible for his or her actions. That would be to accept full-fledged determinism, to argue that a mentally ill person's actions are wholly determined by her mental illness. But there always remains the question of whether she could have acted other than as she did.

On the Kantian principle of 'ought implies can', we should hold people responsible only for what they can do or control. A diagnosis of mental illness tells us only something about the person's ability to control their actions in general; it does not tell us that she could not have done otherwise in this particular case. At most there is a statistical relationship: for example, the probabilistic tendency of certain psychiatric conditions to be associated with criminal conduct, such as depression with shoplifting.[22]

Put another way, Delia's case is not just a clinical or technical question about diagnosis – mental illness, personality disorder or substance abuse? – but an ethical dilemma about whether, even if she is mentally ill, she could still be held responsible for her conduct. We cannot assume a simple causal relationship between mental illness and criminal actions.[23] There are at least two reasons why not. First, even in the case of those who are mentally healthy, there is no simple causal relationship between mental state and action. A sane person could also be tempted to steal a car, but if she does not act on that temptation we do not attribute her law-abidingness just to her good mental health. We distinguish between good mental health and good moral character. Second, and conversely, mental abnormality does not necessarily indicate moral 'abnormality'. Just as even a person with diagnosed mental illness may still be capable of autonomous judgements, such as refusal of consent to treatment,[24] so he may still be able to make considered moral choices.

This brings us into the territory of condition (2), the effect of the agent's desires and intentions upon the action – and also introduces another concept from moral philosophy: *akrasia*, or weakness of will. On the one hand, we want to resist the easy conclusion that mentally ill and mentally healthy people ought always to be treated differently in terms of attributing responsibility. It is consistent, on the other hand, to try to understand the actions of someone who may have mental illness – such as Delia – in terms more conventionally applied to agents whose capacity is not in doubt, but who may not always act according to their better judgements or good intentions.

Akrasia has troubled philosophers since classical times because of its implications for intentionality and rationality. Although most fully discussed in Aristotle, the concept first arises in Socrates' claim that no one knowingly and willingly seeks the greater of two evils or the lesser of two goods.[25] We usually assume that a rational agent intentionally performs X rather than Y because he wants to do X more than Y; so, if he really wants to do Y, what can make him do X?

In the present case, we could magic the problem away simply by saying that Delia is not rational. Akratic action is usually defined as uncompelled, intentional action conflicting with an individual's better judgement.[26] Does Delia have a better judgement? But, first of all, we are not certain that Delia has a mental illness, rather than a personality disorder or a problem of substance abuse.

Secondly, even if Delia is mentally ill, we cannot automatically equate mental illness with irrationality, still less with absence of character – since the mentally ill may be able to demonstrate rationality in some spheres. In the case of Mr C, a schizophrenic detained in a secure hospital was judged competent to refuse consent to a surgical procedure because his ability to deal with personal finances, for example, demonstrated a level of rationality enabling him to understand the consequences of refusal. Susan Hurley advises that 'The general rule is: Attribute irrationality with restraint; be as charitable as possible.'[27] In support of her maxim she cites a warning which psychiatrists are likely to find particularly apt: 'To see too much unreason on the part of others is simply to undermine our ability to understand what it is they are so unreasonable about.'[28]

It is better to treat Delia as having a character, rather than as lacking in character, rationality or moral agency. By treating Delia's actions as akratic rather than necessarily irrational, we accord her a 'privilege' also given to the mentally well. Attributions of *akrasia* are similar in some ways to attributions of irrationality,[29] but not so wholesale. We allow that the mentally well can be weak-willed or inconsistent, too, at certain times. This is less of a blanket judgement than simply calling Delia irrational. And it seems to fit the facts of her case better. We can delineate particular circumstances in which she is particularly weak-willed – with her abusive boyfriend, or after drug use – and when she seems to have some control over her actions – in a hospital environment where staff set firm boundaries. Perhaps her latest episode actually shows some self-awareness and rationality: she knows herself well enough to realize that she has most control over her actions in a secure environment. The 'voices' telling her to get herself arrested so that she can go to prison, or, more likely, back into hospital, are speaking a certain truth. Perhaps she recognizes that she is so frequently weak-willed that this is the best, most rational alternative for her.

We might even say that Delia displays a perverse *strength* of will or character in holding to the course that will get her what she wants – a secure environment – and defending her action in throwing the brick. Similarly, she deliberately sabotages her placement in a less secure environment, overcoming natural revulsion at smearing urine and faeces on the wall in another display of strong will. Whether an action is weak-willed or strong-willed does not depend on its moral content. I can act akratically in *not* performing a wicked or irrational deed that I had already determined to do.[30] Hence Lady Macbeth's reprimand to her husband, 'Infirm of purpose!' (*Macbeth*, II, ii, 52). Akratic action may have a virtuous motive but still be akratic, and seen as such by the agent. Even though Macbeth's hesitations about murdering Banquo are virtuous, rooted in clan loyalty and the duties of a host, he begs to be relieved of them:

> ... Come, seeling night,
> Scarf up the tender eye of pitiful day;
> And with thy bloody and invisible hand
> Cancel and tear to pieces that great bond
> Which keeps me pale!
>
> (III, ii, 45–9)

On the other hand, an agent can also exercise self-control in resisting an immoral action. This commonsense truth leads into such difficulties with the concept of *akrasia* that it might seem better to abandon it altogether. If *akrasia* can be demonstrated both in resisting and in following one's 'better judgement', what use is the concept? In common parlance we get around the problem of *akrasia* by saying: 'I acted against my better judgement'; but this still implies that I was using some other form of judgement, and only introduces further problems about what kind of judgement this could be. There is a risk of infinite regress here.

Perhaps the best course, and the one which best describes Delia's case, involves distinguishing weakness of *will* from weakness of *character*.[31] In deciding on a course of action which conflicts with one's better judgement or good intentions, but sticking with it, it is the latter that is exhibited, not the former. Weakness of character fits Delia's continual failure to make good her promises to Thomas about leading a less disorganized life. It also describes her inability to act according to her better judgement except when made to do so by staff. Again, neither weakness of character nor weakness of will is necessarily the same as weakness of reason: better judgements may be supported by appetites, emotions and all sorts of motives, not just intellect. If we view Delia as weak-charactered rather than as having no character all, the threat to a Kantian analysis of the moral luck paradox recedes.

In chapter 1 I noted that: 'The counsel of despair... would be that luck in character so radically undermines attempts to praise or blame that we cannot really have such a thing as ethics at all.' In fact the greater counsel of despair would be to claim that the possibility of having a character at all is so radically undermined by luck and chance that we cannot really have such a thing as ethics at all. By using the extreme example of Delia Jarrett, I have tested that second counsel and found it wanting. However, I have not fully dealt with the first point. That must await further discussion in chapter 9, on moral luck and genetics.

9

Luck, Genetics and Moral Character

Ronald Dworkin has argued that genetics and genomics threaten to shift the boundary between chance and choice. 'That crucial boundary between chance and choice is the spine of our ethics, and any serious shift in that boundary is seriously dislocating.'[1] Dworkin draws a parallel between the sudden intensification of moral debate brought on by the new technologies in medicine that enabled doctors to 'play God' in extending or curtailing life, and the possibility of a 'similar though far greater pending moral dislocation'[2] occasioned by the mapping of the human genome and the possibility of genetic engineering. We need our genetic basis to be random and beyond human control: hence the popularity of the phrase 'the genetic lottery'. If we can control our genetic inheritance, then we can control too much. 'The terror many of us feel at the thought of genetic engineering is not a fear of what is wrong; it is rather a fear of losing our grip on what is wrong.'[3]

The converse problem, I would argue, is this. Genetics also suggests that we can control *too little*, that in the end we really are not responsible for very much at all – but for different reasons than those suggested by Williams in his enunciation of the moral luck paradox. Behavioural genetics, in particular, raises troubling questions for moral agency. As a Nuffield Council on Bioethics consultative document states:

> One of the central anxieties concerning any biological explanation of human behaviour arises from the belief that we are only morally responsible for those actions that we could have chosen not to perform. In the context of behavioural genetics, the concern is that since we do not choose our genes, then insofar as our genes influence our

behaviour, we are not truly responsible for those aspects of our behaviour: we are at the mercy of our genetic inheritance.[4]

I begin this chapter with a brief preliminary discussion of the vexed question of genetic identity: 'are genes us?' The bulk of the chapter is taken up with cases and discussion illustrating the three particular facets of moral luck which I believe to be most germane to genetics: luck in the decisions that must be faced, luck in antecedent circumstances, and luck in character. Luck in outcomes is, for once, notable by its absence, although it will surface briefly in discussion of luck in antecedent circumstances and luck in character. That does not mean that luck in outcomes is totally irrelevant to genetics: indeed, it might be highly relevant to decisions about individual genetic testing and population screening. However, I have chosen in particular, to spend most of my time on the forms of constitutive luck – luck in antecedent circumstances and luck in character – because genetics brings them particularly forcefully to our attention.

Are genes us?

Even if genes do influence our behaviour, it would be a much stronger assertion – an extreme form of genetic determinism or genetic reductionism – to claim that they constitute our very identity. Yet there is a widespread view of DNA as the modern secular equivalent of the soul – the essence of the person, the guarantor of immortality.[5] If there is some other, deeper substratum than the physiological one, however, then luck or ill-luck in genetic endowment would not necessarily lead to problems of *moral* luck. Our identity as moral agents would remain intact, as would the Kantian notion of the good will. Perhaps our genetic endowment might influence our ability to put our moral decisions into effect, but not the decision-making faculty itself.

A particularly lucid account of the question of genetic reductionism is given by Ruth Chadwick,[6] who locates it within the long-standing debate over what constitutes the person: for example, whether we are our brains. Now, identifying the person with the genome is perhaps more plausible than identifying the person with the brain, which is itself programmed by the genome, as well as by development in childhood. On the other hand, the brain is the seat of self-awareness and consciousness. The point, however, is that both kinds of argument are forms of biological determinism. If biological determinism fails – if what we are as persons is something more than what we are as biological entities – then our identity as persons consists in something deeper, such as our identity as moral agents.

Chadwick begins from a view of personhood as self-awareness, which argues against equating the person with the genome.

> The idea that we could hold up a disk containing our genetic profile and say 'That's me', as has been envisaged by some genome scientists,[7] does not take this into account. On the self-awareness account, it is the capacity to give voice to the statement 'That's me' that is crucial, not the information itself.[8]

If the genetic profile is not sufficient to constitute the person, however, it is certainly a necessary 'blueprint', Chadwick notes – so a weaker form of determinism is suggested. The genome identifies the person in the 'thin' way that a fingerprint does.[9] This would be such a thin account of the person, I would argue, as not to threaten moral agency either. It is true but trivial to say that both Hitler and Mahatma Gandhi were 'created' by the programming in their DNA; that does not mean that we have to say that they were both identical in their moral capacities.

In what sense might the genetic profile be the 'blueprint' for the person? Chadwick reminds us that 'the blueprint metaphor has to be recognized for what it is – a metaphor.'[10] It is one among several competing ways of saying who we are. Furthermore, I would add, even if the blueprint metaphor is the most apt one, construction depends on things other than the blueprint: the quality of the materials (i.e., the quality of health care and nutrition in childhood), the dedication of the workmen (i.e., the parents or other caregivers), and random factors like the weather (i.e., accidents and other environmental factors that affect our development).

A response to this argument, Chadwick notes, might be that, unlike ordinary blueprints, and unlike all the other factors of construction, the genome endures throughout all environmental changes, just as the soul was meant to endure 'throughout all the vicissitudes of life'.[11] But even if genes are the 'essential encoder', that is still not enough to say that we are our genes. Character is determined by many other factors, particularly by relationship to others, and the narrative of one's life cannot be predicted from the outline set forth in our genes. Again, our interactions with others will be influenced by genetic components in our personalities, but not solely by those. In the next two sections I provide data from behavioural genetics, particularly studies of twins reared apart, which show the limitations of genetic determinants of character traits. But even identical twins reared together have different life stories, as Chadwick rightly points out; no one contests that they are separate persons despite having the same genome and even the same mitochondrial DNA, as clones would not.

It is a particularly solipsistic view, I would say, to ignore the impact that others' personalities and actions have on the narrative of our lives. Perhaps a determined genetic reductionist would want to say that others, too, are determined by their genes. But even if that is true in the 'thin' sense, it is another matter to say that the interactions between myself and others are determined wholly by our genes. The whole is greater than the sum of the parts; the interaction cannot be predicted solely from the genetic profile of the participants.

What these preliminary considerations of an extremely complex topic suggest, then, is that the essence of a person and of her character will be influenced but not wholly determined by her DNA; that a narrative approach to character, taking into account the impact of others' characters, is also required; and that the inner notion of moral agency is not necessarily threatened by luck in genetic endowment. These are working hypotheses only; let us examine them further in relation to moral luck.

Genetics and luck in decisions to be faced

The first form of luck I want to consider in this chapter, *luck in the decisions that have to be faced*, raises different questions than the other two, although it is a more common theme in the literature on genetics and medical ethics. In terms of dilemmas about testing and screening, whether there is such a thing as the right *not* to know one's genetic endowment has become a commonplace of ethical discussion, particularly where children are concerned. That the theme is common does not, however, make the decisions any easier. The child's supposed 'right to an open future' translates, in moral luck terms, to a right to avoid facing certain decisions, at least until a later age. The following case study and discussion illustrates these issues.

> Robin Parfit, a girl of fifteen, has recently been returned to her family of origin, together with her ten-year-old brother Alex. Despite protests

from their parents, the children had been placed in care after allegations of neglect and suspected sexual abuse by their maternal grandfather. While the children were in foster care, their father Tom was diagnosed with Huntington's Disease; he had himself tested after his mother died of the condition. At present Tom is asymptomatic, although clinically depressed.

Tom's diagnosis combined with the development of an emotionally abusive relationship in the foster home to increase pressure in favour of the children's return home. Things have been going quite well at home, with the family maintaining a good relationship with Fiona Slattery, the consultant child psychiatrist in the case. Fiona was not involved in the abuse investigation, although she had some involvement in the initial stages of the case.

But now Fiona is uncertain how to respond to Robin's expressed wish to be tested for Huntington's Disease. (The news of her father's diagnosis was broken to the girl by her parents, five months after she returned home, although they have so far kept the news from Alex.) In one sense there is no dilemma for Fiona: the predictive testing guidelines at her local clinical genetics unit stipulate that a patient must be aged eighteen or over to be tested. In the interim Robin can receive genetic counselling, and that process is now under way.

But this raises problems for Robin's long-term management, until she turns eighteen, and risks harming the good therapeutic relationship that Fiona has built up with her and her family. (For Alex, there would be an even longer period to manage.) While Robin is generally a 'laid-back' young woman, she seems quite firm in her desire to be tested now, although being a quiet and compliant sort of person, she accepts what she has been told about the eighteen rule. Her parents also support her right to be tested, not least because Robin has a boyfriend. Robin's mother Sally feels particularly strongly that information should not be withheld from Robin. Sally's older sister has recently developed breast cancer, the condition from which their mother died. Sally is considering having herself tested for the BRCA1 gene implicated in some familial patterns of breast cancer. She has discussed the implications of the test with her husband and daughter.

Fiona wonders whether Robin's request may be mixed with anticipatory grief for her father, with a desire to show solidarity with him. Perhaps she also needs to be the perfect child for her parents, now that she is home from her foster placement. Is she simply too vulnerable, as well as too young, to learn what could be a very ugly truth? A diagnosis of HD in Robin might also sever the bond between her and Alex, or increase pressure for the younger child to be told and tested. Finally, testing could upset the parents' attempt to protect both children from future harm. All these seem important (if hypothetical) considerations to Fiona, but deep down she wonders if she is being paternalistic. Or is it just that she can't endure the idea of knowing for certain that this vulnerable girl carries the Huntington's marker in addition to all her other burdens?

The prior question about luck in the decisions that have to be faced is whether we ought to keep certain vulnerable people, particularly children, from facing them in the first place. It is the common belief that we should which underpins the clinician's dilemma in the case of Robin and Alex.

Guidelines have consistently recommended that the Huntington's test should be 'available only to individuals who have reached the age of majority (according to the laws of the respective country)'.[12] But they have also introduced a potential conflict by noting that 'It seems appropriate and even essential, however, that the child be informed of his or her at-risk status upon reaching the age of reason.'[13] If the age of reason is thought to be younger than the age of majority, is it just that young people should be thought rational enough to cope with this knowledge, but not rational enough to consent to be tested? Robin already knows her at-risk status: she cannot avoid ill-luck in the decisions that have to be faced, the ultimate decision about whether to have the linked marker test for Huntington's Disease. By being denied the right to face the decision now, she is in effect being subjected to further ill-luck, the additional stress of having to do battle for the right to have the test.

Whatever the benefits–harms calculation, adults are allowed to request genetic testing for incurable disorders, subject to limitations of individual protocols, but young people under eighteen are sometimes barred from doing so. Adults are presumed competent to consent to or refuse treatment, whereas children and young people are presumed incompetent unless 'proven' otherwise – e.g., by meeting the standards for *Gillick* competence to consent.[14] Does Robin meet those standards? There is a strong case for suggesting that she does, but it might be objected that she is too vulnerable in several senses – her history of abuse, her recent reintegration into the family, and the very fact that she is at risk for HD.

Yet we are all by definition vulnerable at the time we are asked to give an informed consent to treatment: generally we are ill, or facing uncertain results about a possible diagnosis. Why is Robin any different? There are unique factors in this family's dynamics, one might argue, which could make Robin vulnerable in another sense: vulnerable to parental influence. Is she just trying to show solidarity with her afflicted family? Do her parents have particular reasons for wanting her tested – reasons which are against her individual best interest? If so, we might be entitled to doubt whether her consent meets the crucial legal requirement of voluntariness, and, in ethical terms, whether she is really an independent moral agent.

It may well be true that adolescents are more subject to family influence than adults: studies of fourteen- and fifteen-year-olds asked to make hypothetical medical decisions showed that these teenagers frequently deferred to what they saw as their parents' wishes.[15] But that is just what families are about: studies of adults might equally well show that they did what they thought their spouses or children would want. Again, there is no absolute dividing line between adults and children on the issue of voluntariness of consent or refusal. In *Re T* (1992) a twenty-year-old Jehovah's Witness was compelled to receive a blood transfusion on the grounds that her refusal was insufficiently autonomous, that she was too much under the influence of her mother.[16] Conversely, in *Re E* a judge ordered a fifteen-year-old Jehovah's Witness to receive a transfusion against his wishes, but the boy exercised his right to refuse transfusions when he turned eighteen, and died; his values and beliefs were coherent at fifteen and representative of what they would be at eighteen.[17]

We need to guard against the corollary of distrusting any consent to testing given by an adolescent on the grounds that it 'really' represents pressure from his or her parents. If the young person's values and identity seem reasonably coherent and secure, then a consent should be honoured – as should a refusal. But identity comes only with making choices and having them honoured.[18] It is odd to distinguish between the 'age of reason' at which a young person should be told that she is at risk of HD, and the much later age at which she can consent to be tested. If she is rational enough to know the risks, then arguably she is rational enough to know whether they are real for her. The limbo Robin is in now is doing her sense of efficacy and identity no good at all. In effect it is undermining her moral agency: in the name of protecting her from ill-luck in the decisions that have to be faced, Robin is being subjected to another form of ill-luck. The remaining two forms of moral luck which are implicated in genetics also concern the ways in which the very notion of moral agency is undermined by ill-luck.

Genetics and luck in antecedent circumstances

Luck in antecedent circumstances is the broader of the remaining two relevant forms of moral luck: all our genetic endowment, in a sense, constitutes good or bad luck in internal, rather than external, antecedent circumstances. This seems to leave us terribly constrained by what we are born to be and radically to undermine any sense of human agency. On the other hand, it also imparts a sort of existential freedom: because everything is predetermined by genetics alone, nothing is forbidden by any sort of Kantian universal law. These are radical, foundational speculations that I do not intend to discuss further: their implications are simply too vast for this book.

Our intuitions about luck in antecedent genetic circumstances are confused. We think that being tall is a matter for pride, and being short something to be sufficiently ashamed of for parents to have subjected their children to injections of growth hormone derived from human pituitary,[19] with the terrible ongoing consequences in some cases of Creutzfeld-Jacob's Disease from contaminated injections. We also take pride in musical ability, blond hair, and all sorts of other genetically related attributes for which we can take at best only partial credit. Musical ability may be partially genetically determined, but, as Rebecca West's novel *The Fountain Overflows* demonstrates, innate perfect pitch is not necessarily the mark of the best musician. And then there is always misplaced pride in skin colour. These sorts of confusion are misguided and sometimes serious, as in the examples of CJD and racism. In most of these cases, however, the simple prescription is to discount genetic endowment: we should all be considered equal in our human dignity and value, whatever genotype we are born with. So genetic endowment does not overturn fundamental *a priori* principles such as dignity and justice.

There are other, more medically relevant forms of luck in kinds of genetic endowment: for example, the ill-luck of being born into a family with inherited fatal disorders such as Huntington's Disease or with the BRCA1 and BRCA2 genes implicated in some breast cancers. Again, no major paradoxes are suggested by such cases. The questions that arise, such as whether or not to be tested for the disorder and whether or not to undergo radical mastectomy or other serious procedures, are usually prudential rather than moral, no matter how terrible to make – although in some cases there are ethical questions about how much it is right to keep from other family members.[20]

Where it is a matter of telling children and young people that they may have a susceptibility to a potentially fatal condition, for example, difficult ethical questions clearly do arise.[21] While other decisions about genetic testing and preventative procedures are primarily prudential rather than moral, they are interesting for luck in outcomes, because it is still uncertain that radical mastectomy will prevent occurrence of the cancer, or that the cancer will definitely occur without mastectomy, since the penetrance of the BRCA1 and BRCA2 genes is incomplete.[22] Genetics represents a special case of decision-making under conditions of uncertainty.[23]

However, luck in outcomes is not the main focus of this chapter, so let us return to luck in antecedent genetic circumstances. The difficult cases are those in which ill-luck in genetic circumstances can be seen as leading to morally wrong actions: for example, if psychopathy (personality disorder) were genetically caused, and if a psychopath committed a violent crime, could he be excused as the victim of genetic ill-luck? Can responsibility and moral agency be genetically predetermined? Are some people 'born to be bad'?[24]

Although ill-luck in antecedent genetic circumstances might be thought to excuse unethical behaviour, it is not generally an excuse in law. Attempts to plead diminished responsibility because of genetic predispositions would presumably founder on the same rock as other attempts to prove that a criminal action resulted from a mental disorder. The relationship is merely probabilistic, and we have seen (in the case of the twenty-five prisoners in chapter 3) that the law is not happy about assigning guilt or innocence on a probabilistic basis. Causality cannot be established conclusively by anything short of a one-to-one relationship between (1) having a particular genetic component and being prey to a particular mental illness and (2) having that particular mental illness and committing a particular crime.[25]

In addition there are all the difficulties about whether, even if there were such a thing as a 'psychopathic genotype', it would necessarily be expressed as a psychopathic phenotype – whether someone 'born to be bad' could be saved from being bad by a good environment. With intelligence, the correlation for dizygotic ('fraternal') twins raised together is 0.53, for monozygotic ('identical') twins raised together 0.87, and for monozygotic twins raised separately 0.75.[26] A proportion of the variance in intelligence can be explained by genetics, and another proportion by environment, but, more suggestively for our purposes, neither nature nor nature wholly explains all the variance. That is, differences in intelligence – luck in that particular antecedent circumstance – are not wholly determined by either genetic endowment or home environment: in the case of monozygotic twins reared together, 13 per cent of the variation is not determined by either, or more correctly, by both acting together.

We need to be careful, as ever, not to indulge in genetic reductionism, particularly where simplistic genetic explanations perpetuate inequalities and oppression. The view that men are genetically 'programmed' to be violent or sexually unfaithful, though still stoutly defended by some sociobiologists, is neither good science nor good social policy. And we should be particularly careful where supposed ill-luck in antecedent circumstances, such as the ill-chance of supposedly being born 'more violent' than the other sex, is magically transformed into an excuse for being less rather than more stringent about the extent of one's responsibilities, while at the same time becoming a justification for holding greater power and authority. (Compare the example below of a woman with a family predisposition to alcoholism, who could rightly be expected to be more rather than less vigilant about her drinking patterns.) Where genetic determinism and genetic reductionism are excuses for power and abuse of power, they should be distrusted. As Catharine MacKinnon says of free speech, and as I have written about property rights, when such concepts are used as defences of privilege, they are suspect.[27]

Let us return to the legal parallels. An inventive advocate of the view that genetic endowment entirely determines behaviour might want to make an analogy with the defence of automatism in criminal law. We are effectively sleepwalkers through our own lives if we are entirely ruled by our genome. Automatism is the usual defence to violence or other criminal behaviour committed during sleepwalking, as well as in other patho-physiological conditions such as hypoglycaemia, encephalopathy, epilepsy and post-traumatic states. Since only voluntary acts result in criminal liability, acts over which we have no control, such as offences committed during sleepwalking, should not result in criminal liability.[28] Although the defence of automatism has a certain logic to it, it too is prey to the same problem of causality as the defence of diminished responsibility: the difficulty of establishing with certainty that the physiological condition caused the mental state, and that the mental state directly caused the criminal action.[29]

The reverse could equally well be true: if we are privy to genetic information about our predispositions, we may well be held more rather than less responsible for our behaviour.[30] Someone who has a genetic predisposition to the familial sorts of alcoholism might be expected to be particularly vigilant about her alcohol intake. A large group of studies have confirmed some connection between genetics and alcohol dependence, although there is no one 'alcoholic gene'.[31] Some studies suggest that women are less at genetic risk for alcoholism than men, while others conclude that maternal transmission to daughters is more prevalent than paternal transmission to them.[32] One might conclude that a woman with an alcoholic mother ought to be particularly careful about her drinking, although there are problems here. Since there is no one 'alcoholic' gene, someone who wants to be responsible cannot simply go out and have herself tested for 'the' gene, or even the phenotype, since alcoholism is a classic case of a disease mediated by phenotype, by environment as well as by genetic endowment. The following case of an alcoholic pregnant woman illustrates this interaction.

> Jill O'Mara is a 29-year-old Caucasian with a history of drunkenness, that is, she has been arrested and convicted for drunk driving. Because her mother is a known alcoholic, Jill's teachers wondered whether her learning difficulties were due to fetal alcohol syndrome. She left secondary school at sixteen and has worked intermittently since then. Jill married at nineteen and had a child at twenty; the infant, Jake, tested positive for cocaine and was placed in foster care. Although the social worker has told Jill that Jake is healthy and is doing well in school, she has not been in touch with him or with his foster family. Jill has been separated from her husband Jim for the past two years. Like Jill's father, Jim was a wife-batterer. Jill drinks heavily when she is depressed, which happens especially on weekends, but she rarely drinks during the week when she is working.
>
> Two months ago, Jim returned to town and spent the night with Jill. Some time later, when she realised she was pregnant, she had just been fired from her job. She called Jim to tell him about the pregnancy. Jim said he hoped Jill would get an abortion, but Jill wanted to continue the pregnancy. While searching for a new job, she became increasingly depressed and started drinking heavily. Jim returned and reported her behaviour to the police, alleging that she had placed the fetus in jeopardy.[33]

Are Jill's actions so chaotic, and her character so much determined by her possibly hereditary alcoholism, that she can be said to have lost all moral agency? Does ill-luck in her genetic endowment excuse the risk she may be imposing on the foetus of foetal alcohol syndrome – the same syndrome to which she herself may have been exposed in the womb? If so, should she be restrained forcibly from drinking – as someone who cannot control her own behaviour? Possibly; or possibly others – Jim in particular – are using Jill's supposed inability to control her own behaviour as an excuse for their own wrongdoing. Mary Mahowald, whose case this is, argues that, while the social factors in Jill's life definitely support a diagnosis of alcoholism, we should be very wary of depicting anyone as so entirely at the mercy of genes and social factors as not to be autonomous.[34] That was also my conclusion in the case of Delia Jarrett (chapter 8), where a similar pattern of disorganized behaviour gave rise to the question of whether the worst form of ill-luck in character is not to have anything stable enough to be called a character at all.

Jill's history supports a diagnosis of Type I alcoholism, with a median age of onset of twenty-five years, characterized by psychological dependence and guilt about drinking. Although Type I alcoholism is termed 'milieu-related', it is also thought to have a genetic component.[35] If Type I alcoholism is typified by guilt about drinking, compulsory treatment for possible damage to the foetus is likely only to reinforce Jill's guilt. That possibility, and the argument from Jill's autonomy, has to be balanced against the risk of foetal alcohol syndrome, in this case about 35 per cent.[36] In terms of clinical practice, this is good advice against paternalism; in terms of the moral luck debate, it suggests that we should not be too hasty to view character as determined entirely by luck in genetic endowment or external environment.

On the other hand, Mahowald also warns us against being too quick to accept a libertarian view of Jill's autonomy, which is heavily constrained by both genetic and environmental factors.

> Her probable genetic predisposition to alcoholism and the predisposing social circumstances that she has already experienced are not changeable for Jill. However, her current circumstances could be changed to forestall the phenotypic expression of the disease that threatens her health as well as that of her foetus.[37]

The question is how, and that is a difficult question; however, the focus seems right, insofar as it credits Jill with agency but recognizes that her predisposition towards the disease of alcoholism undermines that agency. As Mahowald continues, 'The nature–nurture debate is settled with recognition that neither side wins, not only because both are inextricably intertwined, but also because a third invisible but real element – the capacity to choose, which allows for moral as well as immoral human behavior – is intertwined with both.'[38]

The difficulty in Jill's case is establishing not just how much irresponsibility to others can be condoned – counting the foetus as an 'other', as a person, for argument's sake – but also how much control Jill has over her behaviour. At a minimum, it seems clear that genetic predisposition does not excuse irresponsibility causing harm to others, although it not clear exactly how much responsibility it requires towards oneself. The parallel in English law would be the case of *R. v. Quick*,[39] where a diabetic who had injected insulin but then failed to eat went into a hypoglaecemic state in which he committed an assault. Recklessness in failing to eat, which is under the diabetic's control, undermines the defence of diminished responsibility or automatism.[40]

Similarly, someone with a genetic tendency to alcoholism might still be held responsible for taking the first drink if she knows that it will be particularly hard for her to resist the second and third – harder than for people who do not have the same ill-luck in genetic endowment. For Jill to return to drinking during the week looks irresponsible, but perhaps only because she had previously shown quite a lot of responsibility in abstaining altogether during the week, while she was working. After all, many people drink both during the week and at weekends without earning themselves a bad name. It is only in contrast to Jill's previously 'supererogatory' behaviour that her current drinking during the week looks so poor. We might want to argue that she should actually be seen as more responsible in giving up during the week than someone with no family history of alcoholism; it is harder for her, and it is more than many people do. On the other hand, she may also know from her own narrative that when she breaks her own self-set limits, such as 'no drinking on weekdays', she does lose control altogether. Although the Alcoholics Anonymous view might hold otherwise, the reason why ex-alcoholics ('recovering' alcoholics) cannot restrain themselves if they take one drink may not necessarily be biological; perhaps it has more to do with their moral agency, which they have demonstrated in setting the limit 'no drinking'. Breaking her own self-imposed rule makes Jill depressed, doubting her ability to run her own life, and the circle continues: she then begins drinking even more heavily.

What Jill's case shows, then, is actually that even extreme ill-luck in genetic endowment and environment does not undermine character so entirely as to destroy moral agency. The point is that even known correlations between physical conditions and wrong actions do not allow us to escape imputations of responsibility altogether. In genetics, *a fortiori*, there is very rarely a simple correlation between a single gene, or even a set of genes, and certain actions. So the depredations of moral luck will be less than they first seem: people can still be held responsible for at least some aspects of their behaviour, even if luck in antecedent genetic circumstances is admitted.

Particularly for a Kantian, who can take refuge in the dictum 'Ought implies can', luck in antecedent circumstances can be circumvented. That is, we cannot be held to duties that are impossible for us to perform, given ill-luck in antecedent circumstances. For a virtue ethicist, luck in antecedent circumstances is both inevitable – the virtues, particularly in classical thought, pertain to a particular social station, so that luck in social station directly determines the virtues to which we can aspire – and paradoxical – virtue ethics therefore has difficulty claiming to be a universally binding moral system. These antecedent circumstances are both external (social class) and internal (genetically determined, particularly by male or female sex, but also externally by the gendered norms attaching to the biological fact of sex). For a utilitarian, luck in antecedent circumstances is relevant insofar as it determines the calculus of probabilities. The chances of my achieving a given outcome may be affected by luck or ill-luck in antecedent circumstances. If responsibility is ascribed on the basis of outcomes, there will have to be some allowable excuses for some agents, whose ill-luck in antecedent circumstances limits their chances of achieving morally desirable outcomes. Inequity in starting positions may be either socially constituted – what Claudia Card calls 'the unnatural lottery' – or genetically determined. As with virtue ethics, this requirement undermines the universality of utilitarianism.

The question of *luck in character* is more specific and more difficult than that of luck in antecedent circumstances, although both are aspects of what Williams calls constitutive luck. If we accept genetic determinism, luck in character becomes a subset of luck in antecedent genetic circumstances. Now of course straight genetic determinism is extremely dubious:

> The probabilistic nature of genetic information, the unpredictability and complexity of multifactorial genetic diseases, the controversies about reliability of some existing tests, and the lack of widely accepted standards for interpreting genetic data make genetic information highly disputable for supporting individual and social decisions . . . Despite the

uncertainty, genetic information is often interpreted under deterministic assumptions on the reliability of its approach.[41]

All the same, even the possibility that character is partially genetically determined leads to difficulties about moral luck and responsibility. Particularly for a Kantian, who emphasizes the hard, jewel-like quality of the good will, luck in character may seem fatally pernicious. Arguably, what Kant means by the good will is different from character, and especially from character as genetically determined: it is noumenal rather than empirical. I think this is a plausible position: as Claudia Card also argues, luck in character is specific to individuals, but the capacity to form the good will is open to all – an attractively democratic aspect of Kant's thought. That accessibility is the basis of human dignity, which is again independent of individual character.[42] Nevertheless, although Card finds much of Kantianism attractive, she maintains that Kant does not devote sufficient consideration to individual differences in character development. As a feminist, she is justly suspicious of universalism that turns out to be gender-specific particularism, and I have also made the same argument elsewhere.[43] So it behoves me to explore a bit further how the possibility of formulating a good will, or any will at all, may be conditioned by character, and therefore by luck.

Gauguin revisited: character, genetics and moral luck

Let us return to Williams's formative example of Gauguin. Williams assumes that the problem about Gauguin's justification lies in the *luck in outcomes* of his decision to abandon his family for the life of a painter, given that he cannot know those outcomes in advance but can only be justified by them. Williams is generally more interested in what he terms incident luck – the justifiability of particular choices – than in constitutive luck, although, because he is also interested in identity, he recognizes that luck in character undermines our ability to assess what outcomes will be right for us. As Card puts it, 'Because who we will become is not immune to luck [for Williams], our knowledge from here of what will be in our interests in the future is limited.'[44] Ironically, however, genetics suggests that our identity is not so malleable as all that, and in that respect lessens the impact of luck on who we will become.

By an interesting coincidence, Gauguin has recently been classified (along with many other artists and poets) as suffering from bipolar affective disorder, or manic-depressive psychosis.[45] This disorder is thought to be partially genetic in origin.[46] If one monozygotic twin has the condition, the other twin's risk of being manic-depressive has been estimated variously at between 70 to 100 per cent, as opposed to 20 per cent for dizygotic twins.[47] If Gauguin was affected by manic-depressive psychosis, and if that susceptibility was genetic, then here is another sense in which Gauguin's moral agency is threatened. Admittedly Williams concerns himself with what he terms a fictional Gauguin, and so if he wished he could omit such considerations, but they are important problems that should be taken into account. Indeed, even if it is not true that the historical Gauguin suffered from bipolar affective disorder, we might want to concoct another fictional Gauguin of our own who did, so as to cover these crucial questions of moral luck in character. Two can play at this game.

Suppose Gauguin left his family not so much with the clear intention of establishing himself as a painter in Tahiti, but simply as some sort of unthinking reaction to either a manic or a depressive stage in his disorder. It might have been the 'high', the hasty decision-making and exaggerated sense of control typical of the manic phase, or it could have been a feeling of unbearable gloom about his Paris life during the depressive phase. The point is that there might be something in Gauguin's character, a mental disorder in fact, that determined his 'decision' to abandon his family. Leaving his wife and children for the life of a painter might not have presented itself to him as a decision at all, still less as a moral one. His sense of himself as a moral agent, and indeed our sense of him as possessing agency, might not have entered into it at all: perhaps he was simply the plaything of his mental illness.[48] If he was subject to a mental disorder, and that mental disorder had a genetic basis, then Gauguin's action was determined in an unsettling way by luck or ill-luck in innate character.

How much character is innate or genetic? The problem that behavioural genetics poses for moral luck is a problem only to the extent that genetics does determine character and behaviour. With the exception of the rare single-gene disorders such as Huntington's Disease and early-onset Alzheimer's Disease, most mental disorders are influenced both by susceptibility genes and by environmental factors, for example schizophrenia and the more common late-onset form of Alzheimer's Disease.[49] However, studies of monozygotic twins reared apart have also yielded substantial correlations in character traits (other than intelligence, mentioned previously): conformity 60 per cent, tendency to worry 55 per cent, aggressiveness 48 per cent, creativity 55 per cent and extroversion 61 per cent.[50] A Danish study hypothesizing a possible correlation between genetic endowment and criminality compared the criminal behaviour of 14,427 adopted men with the criminal records of both biological and adoptive fathers. Although the majority of men with criminal fathers, either natural or adopted, had no criminal record themselves, 20 per cent of the men with a 'criminal' biological father but a 'clean' adoptive father also had criminal records themselves.[51] Another Danish study, of mental illness in adoptees, found a stronger correlation between adoptees and biological parents than between adoptees and adoptive parents, and a particularly high rate in a 'highly creative' subgroup who had achieved national prominence in the arts.[52]

Although the latter finding is interesting in terms of the example of Gauguin, these correlations form a two-edged sword. On the one hand, they suggest that, where an unfavourable trait or a disease is concerned, genetics at most produces predispositions or risks. As I have argued before, genetic factors do not determine all of character or behaviour, and where they do determine it they rarely do so in a straightforward single-gene way.[53] On the other hand, they do suggest that luck in genetically determined character is a consideration, if not the only one. It therefore requires more extensive examination.

While most of the literature on moral luck since the Williams–Nagel debate has focused on luck in outcomes, as the two philosophers do and as my own first edition of this book did, Claudia Card has chosen to concentrate on moral luck in character instead. (Card does not distinguish between luck in character and luck in antecedent circumstances: her focus is really constitutive luck, the combination of the two, and this does create confusions to which I shall return later.)[54] To Card, the Gauguin example is as much about internal luck in character as it is about external luck in outcomes. Gauguin could not know in advance whether he would manifest the character of a great artist. 'The external/internal metaphor for luck is thus misleading. A more relevant distinction is between what is and what is not contingent to our moral agency, regardless of whether it is internal or external to ourselves.'[55]

Card is particularly interested in moral luck and character from the viewpoint of social justice. As in Rawls's device of the 'veil of ignorance', justice is normally thought to require us to forget who we are:

to abstract from the particularities of our own situations, genetically or socially determined as they may be, in the interests of impartiality. And in fact Rawls does deliberately treat intelligence, which we have seen to be partially genetic, as something conferred by chance, rather than as an achievement for which we can rightfully be rewarded. The implication, then, is that justice requires us to transcend good or bad luck in genetic endowment and in character. We cannot claim greater rewards on the basis of good genetic fortune, nor should we be disadvantaged on the basis of genetic misfortune.

However, Card mistrusts the supposed impartiality of this model of justice. Ignoring difference, genetic and otherwise, has its risks:

> A danger of this enterprise is that even were the veil to screen out our knowledge of our histories, it would not thereby inhibit the actual influence of those histories. If anything, the influence of those histories may actually be aided by our very lack of awareness or attention to them. The most successful veils may leave us vulnerable to biases that we are ill-equipped to detect. That is not necessarily a reason to give up striving for the ability to attain the universality that the theory seeks.[56]

Up till now I have been treating luck in character and luck in genetic endowment as problems for ethical theory. Card rightly draws our attention to the ways in which awareness of difference, and hence difference in genotype and/or character, can make us better moral agents, rather than undermine our agency. At least, the opposite – blindness to difference and unanalysed reactions conditioned by our own early history, which we have not yet learned to transcend – does not make us good moral agents. Rather than fearing and denying luck in character, Card seems to suggest, we need to achieve an awareness of the particular limitations and strengths of our individual characters, while still recognizing that there are still certain universal responsibilities that transcend the limitations of genetics and character. This is an attractive notion, and one consistent with feminist models stressing difference.[57]

As moral agents, then, we can actually achieve greater sophistication and consistency in our ethical responses by subjecting them to an analysis that takes luck in character into account. Acknowledging the impact of constitutive luck 'can add depth to our understanding of responsibility and increase our sense of morality's importance',[58] for example by encouraging the virtue of compassion, the realization that 'there but for the grace of God go I'. Dwelling on constitutive luck helps to make individual moral agents better people, Card argues, whatever the conceptual difficulties about the good will and luck in character. By contrast, Nagel feared the effect of moral luck in part 'because the self which acts and is the object of moral judgement is threatened with dissolution by the absorption of its acts and impulses into the class of events.'[59] That is, Nagel's concerns are with the paradoxical and threatening effect of the concept of moral luck, rather than with the benefits for moral development that Card believes an awareness of constitutive luck can bring.

Card makes a clever but somewhat specious point when she notes: 'One thing that makes character valuable is that it prepares us somewhat for contingencies. Fortunately, this does not require that it need not have arisen from contingencies itself.'[60] The problem with this statement is not the double negative: rather it is the way in which Card elides 'character' and 'good character'. The problem of luck in character concerns both 'good' and 'bad' character, but what Card means here is simply 'good character'. As we saw earlier, the greater difficulty arises with 'bad' character or 'weak' character – whatever kind of character is insufficient to form the good will that is impervious to ill-luck in outcomes.

Card's approach is attractive and plausible in many other respects. She is particularly convincing when she argues that taking responsibility for constitutive ill-luck is a crucial step towards the development of moral integrity: that those who have been victims, for example of child sexual abuse, need to avoid the victim mentality if they are to develop as moral agents and mature human beings. This argument is consistent with the views of abuse victims themselves[61] and, more broadly, with recent developments in feminism. However, Card also tends to run together luck in character and luck in antecedent circumstances, and it is really the latter to which her approach pertains.

Where Card is most theoretical, and most interesting in terms of the paradox of moral luck, is in her development of Dewey's notion that we are not born responsible, but become so. To paraphrase Malvolio on greatness, some are born responsible, some achieve responsibility, and some have responsibility thrust upon them. Whereas Williams and Nagel take responsibility as a given, Card argues for a developmental notion of responsibility. (She does concede that Nagel's maxim 'to live in a way that wouldn't have to be revised in light of anything more that could be known about us'[62] is somewhat forward-looking and developmental in its orientation.) Constitutive luck, by focusing our attention on the development of the agent, also draws our attention to the way in which the agent comes to construe and accept responsibility. If this approach is followed, we may find that even those whose genetic endowment severely limits their ability to develop agency and responsibility follow some sort of moral development, even if it is limited.

That style of thought is far less patronizing, as well as far less rigid. As I suggested earlier, someone with a genetic predisposition to alcoholism, who takes steps to guard against slipping into that condition, may even be regarded as morally worthier than the person with no such ill-luck in genetic endowment. So Card's developmental approach to responsibility is promising: it directs our attention to the ways in which agency and constitutive luck can interact productively, without moral agency necessarily being undermined. Furthermore, a narrative or developmental account of responsibility makes us think about ways in which taking on responsibility often gives us further responsibilities, rather than writing them off. As Card says, 'When we have or take responsibility for something that turns out badly, that typically gives us further responsibilities. Since the process of responding to our previous choices (and failures to choose) can go on indefinitely, it may be impossible to say whether a person is "justified" until that person can no longer choose.'[63]

A narrative of choices such as this is far removed from the genetic determinism with which I opened the chapter. Even if genetics shifts the boundary between chance and choice, as Dworkin claimed, that is not the same thing as eliminating choice altogether. The sort of extreme genetic determinism that denies all power of choice is ultimately paradoxical, because I have a choice about whether or not to accept genetic determinism. Genetically 'normed' or determined theories are not only 'counsels of despair',[64] they are also philosophically incoherent. In the final chapter I shall examine another 'counsel of despair' to see whether it fares any better.

10

Moral Luck and Global Ethics

[Non-Kantians] may be disposed to think, so far as morality is concerned, that all that is in question is the pure Kantian conception, and that conception merely represents an obsessional exaggeration. But it is not merely that, nor is the Kantian attempt to escape luck an arbitrary enterprise. The attempt is so intimate to our notion of morality, in fact, that its failure may rather make us consider whether we should not give up that notion altogether.[1]

The question raised by Bernard Williams in this quotation, which was introduced in chapter 1, has not yet been dealt with fully in this book. The aim of this chapter is to remedy that omission.

My strategy elsewhere in the book has been to argue that Williams exaggerates the extent to which the paradox of moral luck threatens the entire notion of ethical systems; that a broadly Kantian approach can survive Williams's critique, which, like Nussbaum's, rests on a misreading of Kant; and that the exit route from the paradox of moral luck involves limiting what agents are responsible for, while retaining the full Kantian notion of agency. Thus, in the case of informed consent, what the thoughtful practitioner is responsible for is allowing as fully informed a consent as possible to develop in the context of the doctor–patient relationship. The more informed that consent is, the greater is the extent to which responsibility for ill-luck in outcomes is transferred, or perhaps jointly shared, between doctor and patient. But responsibility for ill-luck in outcomes does not disappear altogether, and this is right and proper. Otherwise an unhealthy fatalism, an unpleasant paternalism, and a callous or calculating unconcern would come to pervade medical practice. From these ill-effects, patients would have no protection in the law of medical negligence, which, after all, rests on notions of responsibility. My approach, I believe, has the advantage of conforming much more closely to the dictates of medical practice and to the spirit of medical law than does Williams's view, which will strike many clinicians as self-indulgently academic – despite Williams's own distrust of self-indulgence in philosophical argument.[2] I also happen to think that it is theoretically sound, as well as practically useful. Readers who have borne with me up to this point would be surprised to hear that I favoured my position primarily on the consequentialist grounds that it will have a better effect; they need not stand amazed. I do not.

However, although I have argued for my strategy's theoretical soundness on the 'micro' level of examples from applied ethics and the 'meso' level of elucidation of canonical philosophical texts, I have not yet examined the 'macro' level: the radical value pluralism to which acceptance of Williams's position would lead, and the counter-arguments that enable us to think in terms of something which, if not a 'global' ethic, at least gives us the possibility of something like universal standards for judging ethical systems. This is not just an abstract academic question: important notions of human rights rest on such a foundation, and those notions are increasingly important for practitioners, too.[3] This final chapter, then, moves outwards from the practical focus of the preceding six chapters in the sense that it concerns 'global' questions about the possibility of universal ethical norms.

Global ethics is also very much about issues of global justice that cannot be resolved within one nation, such as the duties owed by first-world researchers to third-world populations on whom trials are being conducted. Many of those examples will also raise issues of moral luck. For instance, in a situation of 'equipoise', where there is true uncertainty about which treatment will be more effective, re-searchers may not be able to predict the success of a particular drug in combating a highly prevalent condition whose incidence extends well beyond the trial population. Ironically, this could be seen as a form of ill-luck in outcomes, insofar as it might entail a responsibility for the funders to provide that drug more widely, to the entire population of the country in which the trial has taken place, or even to all develop-ing countries. A national trial in the Gambia, for example, showed that use of bednets treated with insecticide reduced the incidence of child mortality from malaria by about 30 per cent, but the Gambian ministry of health could not afford to provide free insecticide after the trial ended.[4] Should the foreign trial sponsors and researchers have considered it their responsibility to provide ongoing care? Similar issues about the extent of responsibility were raised in trials for reduced doses of zidovudine in pregnant women in Africa to prevent vertical transmission of HIV,[5] in the questions concerning the obligations of the South African and Brazilian governments and the pharmaceutical companies to provide generic antiretrovirals, and, more broadly, whenever vaccines or treatments are developed and tested by developed countries' researchers and funders in the developing world.[6]

Issues about global justice in research are particularly pressing because the organization of trials in the third world by first-world firms often aims primarily to benefit first-world patients.[7] Over 90 per cent of medical research resources go towards developing treatments for disorders responsible for only 10 per cent of the global burden of disease. There has been an increase of over 200 per cent in the numbers of third-world subjects included in new drug trials, and a fivefold increase in the numbers of clinical investigators from the first world working in the third.[8] The choice of research topics is dictated by first-world priorities: with AIDS research, for example, where the virus subtype may differ from one continent to another because of the rapidly evolving nature of the virus, vaccines that may be more useful in less developed countries are often ignored in drawing up research protocols. Although research subjects may benefit from improved health care during the period of the trial, those in the control arm often receive nothing more than the 'best locally available' therapy – often nothing – rather than the standard generally prevailing for first-world control arm participants – either the 'highest attainable' or the 'best currently proven' therapy. Once the trial is over, drugs and vaccines may be made available only to lucrative markets in the first world: for example, vaccine developed from a hepatitis A trial on 40,000 children in Thailand was not made available in Thailand – only to Western travellers. It has been alleged that it is actually in the investigators' interest that there should continue to be a high incidence rate of such conditions as HIV in the developing world.[9] Luck in antecedent circumstances must be conceived on a global scale, at this 'macro-macro level', since globalized clinical research affects the most vulnerable worldwide.

These are important issues in global justice which are coming to occupy the minds of medical ethicists to an increasing extent,[10] but, although applied issues concerning ethical decision-making in the context of economic and political globalization are a crucial component of global ethics, they are not the aspect I want to explore in this final chapter. Rather, I want to focus on the meta-ethical argument that a deep examination of the depredations of moral luck entails radical value pluralism, with disastrous effects for the notion of ethical systems.

Why does Williams maintain that moral luck so radically undermines the foundational notions of morality? The reason transcends luck in outcomes, luck in character, or any of the other sorts of luck that have been identified so far. It transcends luck in outcomes because 'the ideal of morality is a value, moral value, that transcends luck. It must therefore lie beyond any empirical determination.'[11] Without empirical determination of the value of one outcome above another, consequentialism, at least in its utilitarian variant, cannot function, and indeed I argued in chapter 3 that consequentialism cannot provide an adequate response to the paradox of moral luck. However, Kantianism, with its emphasis on the jewel-like splendour of the good will, fares no better, in Williams's view. The ideal of morality 'must lie not only in trying rather than succeeding, since success depends partly on luck, but in a kind of trying that lies beyond the level at which the capacity to try can itself be a matter of luck.'[12] That is, the possibility that there can be such a thing as luck in character, luck in possessing the hard, gem-like pure will, is too much for Kantianism to bear, according to Williams. Whether this is indeed true is debatable. The Kantian conception of the good will is less a character attribute, 'the capacity to try', than an attribute of ethics in itself, of what is required to set up the rules of the ethical game. However, I shall not dwell on this argument, having already defended Kantianism against the moral luck critique more extensively in chapter 2.

But does this argument really undermine the foundations of morality, or only the foundations of two particular schools of morality? According to Williams, there is one further precondition of the moral ideal that is fatally injured by moral luck, and it is this precondition that relates most clearly to the question of value pluralism. As Williams goes on to say, 'The value must, further, be supreme. It will be no good if moral value is merely a consolation prize you get if you are not in worldly terms happy or talented or good-humoured or loved. It has to be what ultimately matters.'[13] To put things another way, the good must in some sense be the ones who eventually inherit the earth, or what is more than the earth. What really matters must be theirs, even if worldly goods are not.

It is only in its own terms, however, that morality can offer these blessings: only to those who are already converted. The language of religion is appropriate, since Williams remarks that the ideal of morality as transcending luck 'is in some ways like a religious conception', although 'it is also unlike any real religion'.[14] The standpoint from which this pure, unadulterated value matters most is the standpoint of morality itself, not that of any particular, or at least modern, school of ethics. (Although Williams also asserts that classical virtue-based notions do not make any such claim, I argued in chapter 2 that this is not so, but at this point I am not concerned to repeat those arguments either.) The moral ideal must claim a transcendent supremacy and universality, in which much of its appeal lies, particularly its security as a bulwark against the depredations of moral luck. However, it can claim that superiority and power only within its own framework, in a circular fashion. As Williams remarks, 'The standpoint from which pure moral value has its value is, once more, only that of morality itself. It can hope to transcend luck only by turning in on itself.'[15]

The crucial corollary is that there can be no such thing as a universal or global ethic, or even the possibility of moral value as being the supreme value in different cultures, although embodied in differing laws, norms and rules. There can be nothing more than moral responses based on personal or group identity. As Williams acerbically notes, those who seek some higher form of justification than that 'have one thought too many.'[16] In fact Williams would seem constrained to argue that even advocates of radical value pluralism have 'one thought too many'. If the very notion of moral value cannot be upheld except from within a moral framework – any moral framework – then there is no alternative to circularity, and even radical value pluralism is caught up in that circularity insofar as it maintains that there are supreme moral values within each culture, or even for each individual agent. If this is true, then it may well be that it is Williams himself who has had 'one thought too many'.

Whether the paradox of moral luck radically undermines the foundational notion of moral value is also akin to the problem of 'rival justices and competing rationalities' posited by Alasdair MacIntyre in *Whose Justice? Which Rationality?* Here is another and rather less radical form of the argument that there is no alternative but value pluralism. The starting point, however, is somewhat different, with no explicit link to the paradox of moral luck. Instead, MacIntyre's case rests on what he views as the circular reasoning by which 'one particular partisan type of account of justice, that of liberal individualism... is later to be used to justify [itself], so that its apparent neutrality is no more than an appearance, while its conception of ideal rationality as consisting in the principles which a socially disembodied being would arrive at illegitimately ignores the inescapably historically and socially context-bound character which any substantive set of principles of rationality, whether theoretical or practical, is bound to have.'[17] There are of course similarities here to Nussbaum's critique of Kant, but those have been dealt with in chapter 2, where MacIntyre also put in a brief appearance. What I want to focus on here in chapter 10 is not the critique of Kantian rationality, but the 'historically and socially context-bound character' of ethical systems. If this premise is accepted, it leads again to radical value pluralism – although not, in MacIntyre's formulation, to the full, incoherent implications of ethical relativism.

MacIntyre depicts a current disastrous state of actual radical value pluralism in the substance of moral beliefs, despite our superficial acceptance of unifying liberal rationality as applied to the procedures by which we adjudicate among them. 'We thus inhabit a culture in which an inability to arrive at agreed rationally justifiable conclusions on the nature of justice and practical rationality coexists with appeals by contending social groups to sets of rival and conflicting convictions unsupported by rational justification.'[18] This dark picture mirrors the opening of *After Virtue*, with its metaphor of an ethical holocaust in whose aftermath we struggle to find anything akin to the old meanings. That holocaust was the Enlightenment and its attendant liberal rationalism.

Although MacIntyre does not frame his critique in such terms, another way of presenting this dilemma is in terms of the current conflict in many Western cultures between liberal democracy and multiculturalism. This is where global ethics enters, construed as ethical questions concerning the possibility of any absolute standards, such as universal human rights. The demand for recognition of ethnic or religious identity seems to enshrine a particular, substantive view of 'a good life', and to go beyond the minimum required for (and indeed the maximum possible in) a liberal democracy – that is, procedural agreement.[19] What unites a liberal society is strong commitment to equal respect for all views and to the procedures established by laws and constitutions to mediate between these views, rather than agreement on what constitutes a virtuous or worthwhile life – which the liberal state cannot and should not determine. But without its own substantive, 'thick' account of the good for humanity, as opposed to its 'thin' notion of procedural justice, modern-day liberalism is poorly armoured against the demands of contending social groups who do possess such notions, even if 'unsupported by rational justification'. However, MacIntyre's project is not to 'thicken' liberalism's notion of the good, but rather to emaciate it further, with a deliberate view towards its eventual death from starvation.

What MacIntyre advocates instead is what the Enlightenment, in his view, has ironically blinded us to: 'a conception of rational enquiry as embodied in a tradition, a conception according to which the standards of rational justification emerge from and are part of a history in which they are vindicated by the way in which they transcend the limitations of and provide remedies for the defects of their predecessors within the history of that same tradition.'[20] This assertion entails the inescapable conclusion that no moral system can be criticized except from within the framework of its own culture, its own historical time and its particular assumptions. That much may appear uncontentious to many readers, but of course it entails deep paradoxes. The claim that nothing can be judged except from within its own culture is presented as being impervious itself to judgement from outside its culture; it holds for all time, supposedly. Yet of course many cultures, particularly religious systems, would entirely reject the claim that their truth is relative. Relativism's incoherence lies in the absolute status of truth that it claims for itself, despite its scepticism about all such absolute standards.[21] Here I merely state the obvious rejoinder to what MacIntyre appears to be proposing.

However, what MacIntyre wants to deny is that this value pluralism necessarily entails total ethical relativism. Each tradition can put its own house in order – although with the apparent anomalous exception of the Enlightenment tradition, whose advocates, long used to lording it over lesser traditions, are hopelessly blinkered, in MacIntyre's view. 'Any attempt to provide a radically different alternative standpoint is bound to be found rationally unsatisfactory in a variety of ways from the standpoint of the Enlightenment itself. Hence it is inevitable that such an attempt should be unacceptable and rejected by those whose allegiance is to the dominant intellectual and cultural modes of the present order.'[22] Liberals' much-vaunted cultural tolerance stops here, it seems. A universal ethical system cannot tolerate a 'radically different alternative standpoint', and its critiques of standpoints such as MacIntyre's own will be entirely coloured by its own prejudices. In one obvious sense this allegation is hardly worth considering: it is simply an illegitimate attempt by MacIntyre to claim that his own argument is unfalsifiable. Whatever arguments are brought to bear against it by advocates of Kantian rationalism are merely an 'inevitable' reflection of Kantians' prior allegiance. On Popperian grounds, that arguments which do not even admit the possibility of their own refutation by any valid means must fail, MacIntyre's attempt to claim that his own argument is unfalsifiable, or at least unfalsifiable by Kantians, is invalid. In another sense, however, it is true that ethical universalism cannot, and, I will argue, need not, tolerate radical value pluralism. I shall come to this counter-argument in the second half of this chapter, but first I want to finish setting out MacIntyre's argument and its relevance to value pluralism.

MacIntyre's value pluralism is in fact less radical than the version set out by Williams. To the criticism that acknowledging the plurality of ethical traditions will mean a babel of ethical systems, each unable to speak to the other, MacIntyre replies with a long and intricate metaphor of how speakers of one language can learn really to think and speak in another, not merely to translate word for word. Absent the metaphor, the point is sometimes expressed in a double negative: 'acknowledgement of the diversity of traditions of enquiry, each with its own specific mode of rational justification, does not entail that the differences between rival and incompatible traditions cannot be rationally resolved.'[23] Neither the metaphor nor the double negative is particularly easy to understand, which is not surprising. Although MacIntyre's value pluralism is less all-encompassing and his despair less profound than Williams's, he is still making a large claim: that from his standpoint 'the problem of diversity is not abolished, but it is transformed in a way that renders it amenable of solution.'[24]

However, it will not be solved by liberal means, even though liberalism is the strongest claimant for universalism, particularly universal human rights. Indeed, in MacIntyre's view, liberalism's failure to solve the problem of value pluralism is *prima facie* evidence that the problem may be incapable of solution.[25] There remains a tension within MacIntyre's thought: he wants to reject the possibility of ethical universals – perhaps exactly because the detested liberalism posits them – but he cannot come up with an alternative that avoids the problem of infinite regress. If 'there is instead only the practical-rationality-of-this-or-that-tradition and the justice-of-this-or-that-tradition', then there is no reason to accept that very statement for anyone from outside MacIntyre's own virtue-centred, Thomist or

Aristotelian preferred traditions. MacIntyre's view that there is nothing but individual traditions arises in the historical context of his disillusionment with liberalism and Kantianism. Why should a liberal or a Kantian, from within their own traditions, accept it as absolute? Presumably MacIntyre's answer would be that the liberal tradition is internally inconsistent, in its failure to present ethical universalism consistently. But this is not an internal inconsistency, rather an externally perceived one as viewed from the virtue traditions. If this is MacIntyre's response to the question of why a liberal or Kantian should accept his claim that there are no moral universals, the reasoning is hopelessly circular.

While rejecting post-modernism and full-fledged ethical relativism,[26] MacIntyre presents residual value pluralism as a realistic strength of his approach, against 'one of the central characteristics of cosmopolitan modernity: the confident belief that all cultural phenomena must be potentially translucent to understanding, that all texts must be capable of being translated into the language which the adherents of modernity speak to each other.'[27] Here perhaps MacIntyre lets his language metaphor run away with him: the resemblance between international English and cosmopolitan, secular liberalism may be only skin-deep. MacIntyre offers no actual evidence of any deeper kinship, whereas it is something of a commonplace in international politics that economic globalization has been accompanied by a surprising resurgence of national and subnational ethnic and religious loyalties, not by cosmopolitanism. Babel's linguistic chaos has not been replaced by a lingua franca on anything but the surface; even if 'everyone speaks English', the fragmentation of deeper loyalties and the pluralism of value systems is not on the wane – arguably, rather, on the increase.

Yet having allowed himself that much free rein, MacIntyre again tightens his own bonds by noting that his task is to find 'some feature or features of a human moral stance which hold of human beings independently of and apart from those characteristics which belong to them as members of any particular social or culture tradition.'[28] If this were really what is required, both radical value pluralism and the contradictions of relativism would be inescapable. To seek to find common features that 'hold of human beings independently of and apart from those characteristics which belong to them as members of any particular social or culture tradition' would be a hopeless undertaking, in MacIntyre's own analysis. Since human beings are morally conditioned by the society and time in which they live, as he claims, any common characteristics they share would be either purely coincidental or dependent on the eye of the beholder. One might say, continuing the language parallel, that all human beings with a certain degree of mental capacity share the ability for language, and that they likewise share the capacity for ethical system-building. This may or may not be true. The point is that, if it were true, it would be trivial. Only humans construct ethical systems, and only humans construct language, let us grant for argument's sake. That of itself does not entail similarities between their ethical systems any more than between their languages. Put more subtly, any similarities it does entail are likely to be coincidental, or even red herrings. English and French share the similarity of having the word 'pain', but only the most superficial observer would assume that the same word carries the same meaning in both languages.

Rather than seeking features which hold of *human beings* universally, it is far more productive, in my view, to seek features that must hold of *ethical systems* generally. This is the Kantian project, of course. Indeed, one might argue that these will be the features that also hold of human beings generally, insofar as human beings are the constructors of ethical systems. Again, this appears at first to be only trivially true. But by shifting the focus from the inductive search for what human beings have in common to the deductive one of what is required for a coherent, universalizable ethical system, we can avoid the incoherence of relativism more effectively than MacIntyre's anti-Kantianism allows us to do.

What a Kantian system also allows us is considerable room for pluralism about what our moral duties are. Although we are bound by the duties generated by the obligation to act on that maxim we could will to become a universal law – one formulation of the Categorical Imperative – these 'imperfect duties leave a lot of latitude.'[29] In the next section of this chapter, I want to say a little more about what sort of latitude that may be, drawing on Onora O'Neill's and Martha Nussbaum's approaches to the sorts of global ethical questions about value pluralism that we have been examining in this section. Whereas Williams, to a great extent, and MacIntyre, to a lesser extent, are value pluralists, both O'Neill and Nussbaum argue in favour of the possibility of certain ethical universals. O'Neill has moved from her previous 'straight' Kantianism towards a bridge to virtue ethics, whereas Nussbaum has done the reverse. I shall present both theorists as more inclined towards Kantianism than to virtue ethics, which may seem a surprise in view of my portrayal of Nussbaum in chapter 2. That is, however, the direction in which her thought has moved since *The Fragility of Goodness*. I shall also argue that this is the direction that must be followed by anyone who hopes to maintain ethical universals against the radical ethical pluralism that the moral luck paradox implies.

Towards justice and virtue: O'Neill's account

I begin, however, with Onora O'Neill's *Towards Justice and Virtue*, a book that can be read on two levels. The first is as an attempt to avoid the sort of warmongering to which MacIntyre often falls prey – for example, in his gratuitous insult to the *New York Times*, 'that parish magazine of affluent and self-congratulatory liberal enlightenment'[30] – and to encourage some form of dialogue between the Kantian and virtue approaches. The second, which follows from the first, is as an effort to maintain some form of ethical universalism, something like a global ethic, in the face of multiculturalism and relativism, so as to provide a secure foundation for universal human rights. In virtue ethics no principle of action has cosmopolitan scope; hence the relevance to ethical particularism versus universalism of O'Neill's attempted reconciliation. A global theory of global justice is the eventual aim, although she says this book only tends towards such an account.

The two levels dovetail nicely, but some caution is called for: the debate about multiculturalism, the second area of concern, is not quite the same as that about universalism, the first topic. For example, liberal political theories agree that the state must be neutral between various conceptions of good life, admitting a certain degree of multiculturalism, but certain virtues can still be required of all (e.g., toleration), and some account of universal morality can still be given. Later in this section I shall develop some of these distinctions further.

My own view is that the core of O'Neill's argument is Kantian, and that it becomes increasingly so as the book progresses. However, she begins with a humbling reminder of the dangers of falling into diatribe on behalf of either camp.

> The results [of this book] may, I hope, seem worth taking seriously both to those who think that human rights are the core of justice, but that there is nothing or little objective to be said about good lives, and to those who think that virtuous characters are the kernels of good

lives, but that preoccupation with obligations and rights is ethically limited and even corrupting. I suspect that, on the contrary, failure to think about justice and virtue in tandem is likely to lead to blinkered and ungenerous, as well as implausible, visions of life, action and politics.[31]

Particularists such as virtue theorists wrongly pass up the chance to say something universal about justice, in O'Neill's view; conversely, universalists unnecessarily deny themselves the opportunity to say something about the virtues.[32] Why, apart from the logical incoherence of full-fledged ethical relativism, should we be concerned to say something universal about justice? O'Neill argues that we actually have little choice: 'Virtually any agent in the contemporary world takes the *scope of ethical consideration* to be more-or-less cosmopolitan for some matters; . . . those whose ethical consideration must be more-or-less cosmopolitan for some matters cannot express it *solely* by means of a mosaic of restricted ethical principles and commitments for dealing with restricted domains of life, but rather must adopt at least some basic ethical principles whose scope is much more inclusive, perhaps more-or-less cosmopolitan.'[33]

Advocates of universal justice may argue against particularism on one or more of these three grounds:

1   Human rights must underpin the virtues (Gewith's view):[34] 'an appeal to local practices and traditions (however venerable, however passionately maintained) cannot but endorse evil practices and traditions, indeed vices.'[35] (O'Neill's own view). (We shall see how Nussbaum has come to accept this criticism of the virtue tradition, largely because of its particular relevance to the oppression of women in some local cultures.) 'Particularist reasoning is intrinsically "insiders"' reasoning. Depending on context, it might be said to be ethnocentric (more flatteringly: communitarian) or simply egocentric (more flatteringly: authentic). Vindication of action is taken not to work across whatever borders there may be between "insiders" and "outsiders": it is reasoning for those who have internalized a given way of thought or life and its norms or traditions, its sensibilities, attachments or commitments.'[36] Therefore particularist reasoning cannot be critical or radical; it is intrinsically *status quo*. Is this what we want of a practical theory of justice?

2   Particularism is inadequate in the contemporary world. One way of phrasing this point might be to note that particularism erects

no barrier against economic and political globalization[37] and affords no way of dealing with the sorts of applied ethical questions of global justice arising in the context of globalization that we met at the start of the chapter. O'Neill's preferred formulation, however, is that complex modern states must be universal within their boundaries, and indeed across national boundaries, because international economic systems are also complex. Particularism by itself is therefore hopelessly nostalgic.

> A particularist account of ethical relations and reasoning that might have been practically adequate in a world of homogeneous, closed societies will almost certainly prove practically inadequate in a world marked by cultural pluralism within states, vastly intricate interregional, international and transnational relationships, and constantly shifting patterns of integration and connection between different spheres of life and different social groups. Far from being sensitive to the ethical pluralism of modernity, particularists are largely blind to it, since they see ethical life as encapsulated in distinct domains by rigid grids of categories and sensibilities. From the perspective of their critics, particularists who ground restricted ethical principles in 'our' traditions indulge a cosy but dangerous nostalgia for a world now lost, and refuse to engage with the world we actually inhabit.[38]

Not only is the 'traditions' approach nostalgic; it is also naïve in its assumption that preserving local traditions is somehow democratic. (One might adduce the case of the 'Asian values' ideology used to underpin undemocratic regimes in Singapore and Malaysia.) But actually communitarianism is less democratic and more advantageous to political elites than cosmopolitanism, which is discredited by its association with neo-colonialism but which actually offers greater popular accountability. 'In a post-imperial world, cosmopolitan arrangements threaten rich states with uncontrolled economic forces and immigration and demands for aid for the poor of the world, and autocratic states with demands that human rights be guaranteed across boundaries.'[39]

3   Even if particularist principles could resolve conflict, there is still no reason for thinking them ethically authoritative. Something more basic *is* available, although particularists insist that there is no way for an individual or community to 'go behind' justification in terms of identity or traditional practice. We have seen, however, that, at least in MacIntyre's formulation, the most we can expect is for

individual traditions to put their own houses in order, making them internally coherent. There is no reason for proponents of any particular value system to accept external principles inconsistent with that system's own logical grounding, just as there was no reason why Kantians should accept MacIntyre's view – a view from outside, and not a view from nowhere, in Nagel's characterization of the neutral ground that MacIntyre rejects.

Nevertheless, O'Neill cautions against assuming that universalism must be alive and well merely because particularism's health is less than perfect. Although most of the account is more universalist than particularist, accommodating the latter to the former in a rather one-way manner, at the end of her first chapter she concludes:

> The unexplained divergence in the way the two domains of ethics are now discussed may reflect the mere reality that neither is firmly anchored. It has been tempting to continue to think of justice in universalist terms, because the broad scope and close-to-cosmopolitan tasks of justice are so important in the modern world. It has been tempting to think of virtue in particularistic terms because other approaches seem not merely unavailable but questionable in a culturally diverse world. If the crisis of foundations is to be taken seriously, there is little to be said for succumbing to either temptation. There is little to be said on behalf of inclusively universalistic principles, including those of justice, unless they can be based on convincing practical reasoning, which either sustains or replaces justifications once based on metaphysical or religious certainties. There is little to be said on behalf of particularist conceptions of the virtues unless convincing reasons are found, which show why appeals to shared traditions or to individual sensibilities justify ethical claims.[40]

This warning seems singularly apposite to particularisms that claim to be universalisms. I have argued elsewhere, in my *Property, Women and Politics*, that many canonical theories of property and justice typically exhibit just that fault, although they may contain concepts that are potentially appropriate to thinking about women's liberation if developed, as I attempt to do, into genuinely universal notions that count women in.[41] Feminist theory offers the resources and the pedigree to help settle the universal–particular debate in global ethics, and in the concluding sections of this chapter I shall return to the parallels between feminist post-modernism and radical value pluralism, arguing that both are counter-productive and incoherent. What can be substituted for them will, I hope, become clearer at that stage of the chapter. For now, let us return to O'Neill.

So far we have been examining O'Neill's claim that ethical particularism, in particular virtue theory, wrongly passes up the chance to say something that must be said about universal justice. The other half of O'Neill's earlier assertion was that universalists unnecessarily deny all of particularism, depriving themselves of the opportunity to use the virtues of the virtues. In O'Neill's partial compromise with particularism, some practical reasoning must have universal scope, although some can be permitted to have particularistic scope, provided that it is 'followable' by all within the relevant wider community. Special pleading by particular communities can be allowed on a procedural basis, rather than a substantive one, so long as all, including outsiders, can follow the rationale. Note the contrast to MacIntyre's emphasis, which lays stress on improving the coherence of an ethical tradition's narrative as read by its followers, but which, despite the elaborate linguistic metaphors of translation, does not include any such specific requirement as O'Neill's demand that outsiders to the tradition should be capable of following its rationale. 'For example, the conditional claims of particularist reasoning that has its place in a restricted context might gain sense and authority in the eyes of a far wider audience not because – as it happens – all those in the more inclusive domain came to hold the relevant restricted beliefs or norms, but because wider reasons could be given for viewing the actual beliefs and norms of the more restricted context as ethically significant.'[42]

O'Neill's conception of wider reasons is rather similar to the notion of procedural legitimacy in political theory: subgroups within a polity may disagree on substantive policies, but they can agree to abide by the procedures set up to adjudicate between them, as when the losing party in a UK election becomes the 'loyal' opposition. 'Followable' means both intelligible to this wider audience, in the Kantian sense that the particular principle's adoption by the wider community would not be logically incoherent, and, more stringently, capable of being acted on, offering real possibilities for living in this world. This rules out the idealized autonomous individual beloved of principlist medical ethics, among others:[43]

> Reasoning is defective when reasons misjudge or misrepresent what others can follow. For example, one of the many uses of idealized conceptions of the person is to obscure the realities and vulnerabilities of others, and so obscure the fact that the purported reasoning is simply

inaccessible to some for whom it is disingenuously said to provide reasons for action.[44]

I would interpret O'Neill's formulation as also ruling out an ethic which offers women no scope for action, nothing to act on, no status as moral agents: such an ethic is therefore illegitimate, even if it is intelligible to them as part of a traditional set of norms.

The result is a minimalist collection of universally agreed principles that gives reason to doubt extremely comprehensive catalogues of human rights, which are both too prescriptive – leaving little space for those ethical particularisms that meet the toleration test – and so vast as to be impractical.[45] This slant, too, is Kantian, consistent with the argument I make elsewhere, that we must limit what agents are responsible for but can hold them fully responsible, imperviously to the operations of luck, once we have done that. As Kant says in the *Critique of Pure Reason* of the modest outcome of his universal ambitions in constructing a system of practical reason:

> Indeed, it turned out that although we had in mind a tower that would reach the heavens, yet the stock of materials was only enough for a dwelling house – just roomy enough for our tasks on the plain of experience and just high enough for us to look across the plain. The bold undertaking had come to nothing for lack of materials, quite apart from the babel of tongues that unavoidably set workers against one another about the plan.[46]

But the point is that we do have somewhere for us all to live, a moral system constructed on our measure and for our modest comfort. Like Thoreau, we may actually be more content in the little cabins that we construct according to our own plan. In a passage that both echoes and refutes MacIntyre's language metaphor, O'Neill argues that universalistic ethical reasoning can provide such structural plans that can be followed across a range of cultures, yet may also allow considerable diversity of design. In contrast, to the extent that particularistic traditions ignore the dictates of universal reason, the resulting incomprehension among contending accounts of rationality and justice means that 'only the Tower of Babel can be built.'[47]

> Practical reasoning that seeks to give an account of the ethical constraints, the lives and forms of life – the 'buildings' – that can be made out of available materials must start from sober considerations of the

real possibilities for those who are to build and to live with what they have built. They must meet the condition of being followable by those for whom the reasoning is to be relevant. These starting points set a task rather than provide a solution...I shall argue that (fortunately) they do not provide enough to regiment what can be built: an amazing variety of lives and forms of life can be built within these constraints; but also that (equally fortunately) they require action to meet certain identifiable standards. Would-be builders who observe the constraints of reason will find that these *partly* shape the 'buildings' they can produce, while those who try to ignore them will find that some others think some of their proposals for action baffling, arbitrary and unfollowable. When the constraints of reason are ignored, coordination and communication fail: only the Tower of Babel can be built.

Nussbaum and the capabilities approach

O'Neill's approach represents one form of compromise between universalism and particularism, achieved primarily through concessions from Kantianism to virtue ethics. Martha Nussbaum's recent work, grounded in the 'capabilities' approach originally developed by Amartya Sen, demonstrates another, achieved by movement in the opposite direction. The 'capabilities' approach is intended to provide the philosophical justification for global ethics in distributive justice, 'a bare minimum of what respect for human dignity requires'.[48] Nussbaum's project is to 'identify a list of *central human capabilities*, setting them in the context of a type of *political liberalism* that makes them specifically political goals and presents them in a manner free of any specific metaphysical grounding.'[49] The list of capabilities is of course open to question, and indeed Nussbaum herself has altered it from earlier versions, now giving greater importance to property rights.[50] She does not develop her arguments about property at any length, however, and in this she implicitly accepts the usual stereotype, common even among feminists, that women can only be objects of property rather than subjects.[51] For the purposes of this chapter, however, the more important question is whether it is possible to develop a universally agreed set of capabilities, 'free of any specific metaphysical grounding' and immune to problems of philosophical relativism.

Nussbaum presents these capabilities in an Aristotelian manner, as those essential to human flourishing. Far from avoiding questions of relativism, of course, an Aristotelian approach invites it, insofar as the qualities or virtues appropriate to flourishing are culture-specific. Nussbaum needs an account of what it is to be human that overcomes such cultural relativism, but too much rests on rhetorical terms such as 'dignity', 'human' and 'flourishing'. This becomes clear if we substitute 'dog' for 'person' and 'canine' for 'human' in this sentence: 'Beneath a certain level of capability, in each area, a person has not been enabled to live in a truly human way'.[52] To say that such-and-such a capability is 'human' means little in normative terms: the capability for violence is also human, although most of us think it should not be encouraged, but rather fettered. Nussbaum might counter that she has further specified that these capabilities must be 'informed by an intuitive idea of a life that is worthy of the dignity of the human being'.[53] But of course many warrior cultures, including the ancient Greeks, have viewed violence in war as the very essence of the dignity of the (male) human being. Nussbaum admits that her notion of dignity is intuitive, but intuitions are largely culture-specific. We cannot get there – the idea of a global ethic, particularly one respecting women – from here – a naturalistic argument. Nussbaum is good at deconstructing arguments rooted in cultural relativism, as in her first chapter, but she is less successful in providing a universalistic alternative to limit what she terms 'the intolerance of cultures'.[54]

In fact the argument does not remain Aristotelian for long: Nussbaum borrows a great deal from liberal thought, in particular from the version found in John Rawls's *Political Liberalism* (1996). Here she edges over into a rights-based approach, although she also argues that the capabilities approach has the edge on rights because it is not uniquely identified with the Western tradition. Distancing herself from Aristotle, she characterizes her own proposal '(clearly, unlike Aristotle's) as a partial, not a comprehensive, conception of the good life, a moral conception selected for political purposes only'.[55]

Here we come down to questions of strategy. Nussbaum does recognize that other, non-Western cultures also have conceptions of human rights,[56] and there I think she is correct. The Zimbabwean academic lawyer Charles Ngwena and his South African colleague Michelle Engelbrecht, for example, have described something which sounds very much like human rights as being found in traditional South African law, the concept of *ubuntu*, which they explicitly identify as being compatible with a Kantian, deontological ethical system. '*Ubuntu* signifies the recognition of the human worth and respect for the dignity of every person.'[57] In *S. v. Makwanyane*, Mokgoro J said this about the meaning and concept of *Ubuntu*:

> Generally, *ubuntu* translates as humaneness. In its fundamental sense, it translates as *personhood* and *morality*. Metaphorically, it expresses itself in *umuntu ngumuntu ngabantu*, describing the significance of group solidarity on survival issues so central to the survival of communities. While it envelops the key values of group solidarity, compassion, respect, human dignity, conformity to basic norms and collective unity, in its fundamental sense it denotes humanity and morality. Its spirit emphasises respect for human dignity.[58]

Might it not be a better strategy to concentrate on appealing to those existing concepts of rights in non-Western cultures, rather than playing into the hands of anti-feminists whose intuitions are rather different from Nussbaum's own? Why concede ground to what Nussbaum describes as a mistaken belief?

That would be the political argument against Nussbaum's capabilities approach; the philosophical one is that a *description* of human capabilities cannot generate *normative* rules without appealing to some prior ethic, probably either a Kantian or a rights-based one. What is so special about being human? Presumably it is that we have practical reason and the ability to set up reciprocal, binding moral and political systems, which entail notions of contract and rights. Nussbaum implicitly concedes this point when she notes: 'Not all actual human abilities exert a moral claim, only the ones that have been evaluated as valuable from an ethical viewpoint.'[59] Further, she concedes that 'capabilities as I conceive them have a very close relationship to human rights',[60] but goes on to say that the capabilities approach is preferable because it is clearer. Although I agree that there is a great deal of well-meaning but slipshod use of rights language, I hope that I have given sufficient cause to doubt whether the capabilities approach, in Nussbaum's formulation, really is any clearer.

On the whole, then, I think that O'Neill's response to the problem of value pluralism is the more cogent and coherent. What is interesting in both responses, however, is that each claims with some degree of success to refute Williams's critique of moral luck as entailing irresolvable value pluralism. Another way of framing this debate, and of responding to Williams, requires us to go outside the frameworks of mainstream philosophy and into feminist theory's parallel debates concerning identity, essentialism, particularism and difference. This is what I shall endeavour to do in the final section of this chapter, and of the book.

The final synthesis: feminism, global ethics and moral luck

Nussbaum is leading us in the right direction when she suggests that we need to look to feminism in resolving the question of whether a global ethics is possible, but she is right for something less than the right reasons. Certainly the oppression of women matters, and it matters whether a relativist ethic cannot find the right weapons against that oppression. But it is within the theoretical debates in feminism, with which Nussbaum appears unfamiliar, that we can find some glimmerings of a larger answer to the question.

At the beginning of this chapter I raised the possibility that Williams's view of moral luck as entailing radical value pluralism is effectively hoist with its own petard. Caught in an inescapable circularity, Williams's argument entails the disintegration of practically everything, including itself. The very notion of moral value as the supreme value, which is after all what makes it moral value, can no longer be upheld, even if we confine it to 'the supreme values of one culture' or 'the supreme values for each individual'. In other words, the very notion of value slithers away if the paradox of moral luck is taken seriously enough, Williams argues. I have shown elsewhere in this chapter how other philosophers attempt to stem this disintegration from within Kantian or virtue frameworks, or from a marriage of the two (O'Neill and Nussbaum). MacIntyre, on the other hand, steps outside the boundaries of philosophy into linguistics, drawing on language metaphors to argue that we can at the very least speak clearly within our own moral languages. That stratagem seemed less than successful, however.

If we remain within the boundaries of philosophical analysis, but turn instead to feminist theory, something strange yet eminently predictable occurs. The debates that now exercise mainstream philosophy, international relations and political theory so vigorously, concerning universalism, particularism, cosmopolitanism and the possibility of global ethics, have already been going on in feminist philosophy for at least twenty years, almost entirely unremarked by 'canonical' philosophers.

In debates concerning post-modernism, deconstruction, identity and difference, there has emerged the risk that the very notion of 'woman' may slither away, making it impossible to develop a feminist politics. This tendency is particularly pronounced in the work of Judith Butler and Luce Irigaray.[61] Irigaray's view resembles Butler's insofar as both present a self in interior conflict, a disunited subjectivity; both rely on the insights of psychoanalytic theory, particularly of Freud and Lacan, in putting unresolved and unsymbolized desires to the fore. The psychoanalytical model directly challenges the view of the self as unified moral agent and thus builds in additional ways in which moral luck can undermine the very notion of moral agency. Not only is the possession of the correct character traits to produce the good will possibly a matter of luck: the possession of anything like unified character is utterly undermined.

Although moral luck is rarely mentioned in the same breath as this model of disjointed subjectivity, least of all by Butler or Irigaray themselves, this is one reason why it is interesting to compare the moral luck debate with current feminist theory, but it is not the principal one. The main point is that the tension around whether there can be such a thing as a subject, and the corollary practical implications for feminist politics of admitting that there might not be, parallels the disintegration of the moral life if we accept Williams's arguments, with practical implications for global human rights and the question of whether there can be such a thing as global ethics. The identity of the subject has of course been a matter of concern in mainstream philosophy since Locke's time, at least, but there is no parallel in mainstream philosophy to the manner in which feminist deconstructionism has been seen to be in conflict with more essentialist feminisms, concerned to preserve the notion of 'woman' in order to retain the necessary political and conceptual apparatus to fight the oppression of women.

Feminisms such as the 'genealogical' models proposed by Butler and Irigaray doubt whether there is such a category as the subject at all, as distinguished from 'interpretation' feminisms which enhance women's status as subjects by stressing their unique experience and voice.[62] Here is a clear parallel with Williams's doubts about whether there can be any such thing as the supremacy of moral values over all other sorts of value, and thus whether there can be such a thing as ethical systems, insofar as ethical systems typically claim to concern the highest things. (I interpret religious systems as a form of ethical systems, consistent with my broadly Kantian approach.) Furthermore, critics of genealogical models argue that deconstructionist feminism is parasitical on the very claims it seeks to unfound, and that this is particularly true in its questioning of the self.[63] Only a subject can engage in the sorts of deep doubt about subjectivity to which the work of Butler and Irigaray gives voice, for elementary Cartesian reasons. Similarly, I would argue, only a moral agent, and a serious-minded one at that, can engage in the sorts of deep doubt about moral luck and the abolition of the entire notion of moral systems to which Williams's work calls us.

Without a unified category of 'woman', there can be no political impetus towards the ending of women's oppression, which I take to be the definition of feminism.[64] A feminist deconstructionist therefore seems to be trying to make herself disappear. In Williams's instance, a moral philosopher who doubts the possibility of moral philosophy is doir.g much the same. If moral luck is as all-encompassing in its destructive effects as Williams claims, it cannot claim to be 'moral' luck, because there can be no such thing as 'moral'. Yet it is the moral power of luck that undermines the whole of Williams's argument – its power to awaken remorse and regret, the manner in which its distribution among people's characters is not merely a neutral fact, such as the distribution of green eyes or ginger hair. The positive aspect of feminist deconstructionism, however, has been the manner in which it has drawn attention to the possibility of a subjectivity that women can actually own, rather than one borrowed from male psychological development. While Irigaray, for example, is often seen as one in a chain of post-modernist and post-structuralist attempts to deconstruct the subject, she is actually more concerned to create a subjectivity that women can own. Since women have been deprived of an appropriate symbolic by psychiatric theory rooted in male experience, 'they have never had a subject to lose.'[65]

In other words, what is suggested for global ethics by a modified feminist deconstructionism, and by feminism more generally, is this: there can still be ethical systems, and ethical universals, but they must be truly universals. They cannot be particularist theories masquerading as ethical universalism. Much of modern feminist theory, particularly such powerful critiques of liberal democracy as Carole Pateman's *The Sexual Contract*, was concerned in its early days to demonstrate with great perspicacity exactly how shaky were the claims to universalism of the liberal concepts of political selfhood: citizenship, contract, property and rights. Later feminist work has been concerned to reconstruct those concepts to make them genuinely universal, incorporating women's experience as well. In this camp I count my own work on property, together with feminist theories of the state (Catharine MacKinnon), political obligation (Nancy Hirschmann), democracy (Anne Phillips), justice (Iris Marion Young) and authority (Kathleen Jones). Rather than jettisoning these foundational concepts of moral and political theory altogether, or denying the very possibility that there can be foundational and universal concepts, feminists have sought to rebuild them on a firmer footing. Whereas earlier second-wave feminism typically rejected canonical political concepts as implacably oppressive to women, there is now much more optimism about reconstructing them to make them work for us. The reworking of these concepts by women of colour is also important (for example, by the authors in Toni Morrison's collection *Race-ing Justice, En-gendering Power.*) Similarly, concepts of women's rights have been incorporated into mainstream development ethics, but tailored in such as fashion as to enable some sort of accommodation with important aspects of traditional cultures.[66] Such accommodation is never easy, but it is practically necessary and theoretically revitalizing.

What does this possibility from feminism offer global ethics? Of particular importance has been the way in which feminist theory increasingly combines universalism and difference. Denying that so-called impartialist theories of justice are truly universal, Iris Marion Young, for example, offers a paradigm that can also be applied to the question of whether there can be global theories of justice.

> Universality in the sense of the participation and inclusion of everyone in moral and social life does not imply universality in the sense of the adoption of a general point of view that leaves behind particular affiliations, feelings, commitments and desires. Indeed ... universality as generality has often operated precisely to inhibit universal inclusion and participation.[67]

The parallel in global ethics will be a concern with inclusion and participation, at the expense of any attempt to create a single set of global principles. Young might well dismiss such attempts to transcend difference as imbued with 'the logic of identity', as she does with Rawls's account of justice. Whereas 'the logic of identity ... constructs totalizing systems in which the unifying categories are themselves unified under principles, where the ideal is to reduce everything to one first principle',[68] the politics of difference does not seek so relentlessly to reduce all differences to unity. On one level, what Young offers is a rather 'thin' account of global justice, one concerned more with procedure than with substance. On the other, however, her account is deeper, if not 'thicker', than principlist accounts that seek to unify disparate global experience into a single framework. Difference is foregrounded in Young's account of justice, but the proselytizing power of injustice is not 'relativized' out of existence. Indeed, she would argue that opponents of oppression are in a better, more realistic position if they employ a transformational rather than an assimilationist model, if they take difference into account rather than attempt to impose a single model of justice with no respect for group identities.

At a minimum, global ethics can take a warning from feminism against both Williams's despair about the foundations of ethics itself and the dereliction of duties to help on a global scale that can be occasioned by an over-concern for cultural tolerance. The Indian feminist Uma Narayan offers cogent illustrations of the latter phenomenon in her book *Dislocating Cultures: identities, traditions and third-world feminisms*. Well-intending Western feminists, Narayan argues, are too ready to concede toleration to non-Western practices that oppress women; they are crippled by their own guilt, as members of the Western elite that benefited from imperialism, colonialism and neo-colonialism, and which continues to benefit from economic globalization. They are too quick to abandon the possibility of a global ethics that genuinely works for women, and too prone to dismiss third-world feminists who actually agree with them on its foundational principles of equal gender justice. When Narayan mentions her opposition to *sati*, female genital mutilation, or sex-selective abortion, for example, she is usually met – even by feminists – with the accusation that she is too Westernized to be an authentic voice of Indian women. The only acceptable role for Indian women, she feels, is as oppressed victims.[69] Mired in their own discouragement and stereotypes, Narayan accuses, together with their doubts about the very category of woman, Western feminists too readily ignore what is really a very simple matter of justice, and a call for help. Similarly, Susan Moller Okin has warned first-world feminist theorists not to ignore, in their own preoccupation with difference, the reality of sameness of circumstances in reproductive health, poverty, legal rights and other areas for many women across the world.[70]

The same can be said of global ethics. Whether or not meta-theoretical agreement can be reached across cultures and religions is less relevant than the areas on which agreement can and should be possible. This is indeed the approach taken by Nussbaum in her capabilities approach, and it is indicative that, although the theoretical origins of that approach are somewhat bastardized, what it calls for, in terms of redistributive justice, meets with agreement from both Western feminists such as Nussbaum claims to be and Indian grassroots organizations. The top-down, unifying approach to global ethics, seeking agreement on foundations across cultures and religions, is in this sense both less productive and less helpful than the bottom-up approach seeking agreement on concrete reforms and practical issues rooted in women's experience – what Alison Jaggar terms 'feminist practical dialogue'.[71]

If we cannot reach agreement on whether there can even be such a thing as ethical values, we are even less likely to attain the top-down, meta-theoretical sorts of agreement. If we feel we must attain the top-down kinds of agreement before any practical reforms are possible, we simply can't get there from here. This is another sense in which Williams's view is self-indulgent. I have also argued that it is philosophically incoherent; but, even if it were analytically sound, we would have reason to distrust its practical implications. Thankfully, things really are much simpler than that. The extremes of distribution which have been exacerbated by debt and economic globalization are *so* extreme that the practical implications are difficult to ignore. Equally simple is the sameness of human suffering: as Rosemarie Tong puts it in relation to a global bioethics,

> We all experience pain, suffering and death; and since we are all equal in this way, it is the task of health care to serve each of us as if we were the paradigm case of treatment for everyone. Feminist bioethicists are among the leaders in the movement to make health care attentive to people's *differences* so that it can help people become the *same* – that is, equally autonomous and equally the recipients of beneficent clinical practices and just health care policies.[72]

Feminism has transcended its own crisis of faith – similar to Williams's profound doubts about the possibility of ethical systems, eroded by moral luck – to incorporate notions of difference into a programme of political action. For example, standpoint feminisms[73] question the notion of the 'view from nowhere' as a prerequisite of ethical systems, drawing strength from the different perspectives of oppressed groups as enhancing the accuracy of supposedly universalist formulations.[74] Whereas, 'typically, philosophical theories of justice have operated with a social ontology that has no room for a concept of social groups', Young argues that only a concept of justice that begins with the concepts of group domination and group oppression, attending sensitively to real social differences, can succeed in social reform.[75]

Thus second-wave feminism has overcome its initially inward-looking, psychoanalytical fixation on difference and disjointed subjectivity to reaffirm the possibility of struggle against injustice, enhanced by a realistic incorporation of difference where difference really is something more than an excuse for inaction. This is the counsel of action, rather than despair, that feminism can teach global ethics. Its concentration on group identity mirrors only superficially Williams's own conclusion from the paradox of moral luck, that in the end there is nothing but the identities of groups and cultures. The politics of difference is in one sense compatible with Williams's own conclusions, but such scholars as Young would perhaps criticize Williams for accepting the notion of a 'ground zero' of impartiality as the only basis for ethics. If that 'view from nowhere' is not available, as Williams argues, due to the depredations of moral luck, that does not necessarily entail radical value pluralism or the political quietism that inevitably accompanies total relativism. Feminism's version of difference is not quietist but reformist: it does not view all such identities and norms as equally valid, nor does it seek to return to a communitarian or classical golden age, as Williams has tended to do in his work since 'Moral luck'.

To put this point in the Kantian terms for which I have argued throughout the book, our imperfect duties leave us a great deal of latitude, but we have a strict obligation to carry out those duties which we do take on. To put the matter in feminist terms, these duties will include working to minimize oppression against women, but how that oppression 'shakes down' will include both commonalities and differences across cultures. If we can hang on to these two basic precepts, we will find the paradox of moral luck does not undermine the foundations of ethics; rather, it draws our attention to what we can sensibly hope to achieve.

Notes

Chapter 1   Ethics versus Luck?

1   Daniel Statman, 'Introduction', in Statman (ed.), *Moral Luck*, p. 1.
2   Statman, 'Introduction', p. 2.
3   Immanuel Kant, *Fundamental Principles of the Metaphysic of Morals*, first section, third paragraph, cited in Thomas Nagel, 'Moral luck', in *Mortal Questions*, p. 24.
4   Martha C. Nussbaum, *The Fragility of Goodness: luck and ethics in Greek tragedy and philosophy*. Two lengthy critical reviews are sceptical of Nussbaum's claim, regarding it as anachronistic: John M. Cooper's article in *Philosophical Review* and Nicholas P. White, 'Rational self-sufficiency and Greek ethics'. These criticisms, along with Nussbaum's work, will be discussed in greater detail in chapter 2.
5   Bernard Williams, 'Moral luck', p. 24.
6   Bernard Williams, in *Proceedings of the Aristotelian Society*, supplementary volume 50 (1976), pp. 115–35; Thomas Nagel, reply to Williams in the same volume.
7   A recent literature search on Bioethicsline, using the search term 'moral luck', revealed only four entries, three by myself! – including the first edition of this volume, *Moral Luck in Medical Ethics and Practical Politics*. The remaining citation was Margaret Urban Walker's 'Geographies of responsibility'.
8   Judith Andre, 'Nagel, Williams and moral luck'; Michael Zimmerman, 'Luck and moral responsibility'; Walker's 'Geographies of responsibility'; the authors in the volume *Moral Luck*, edited by Daniel Statman; and Statman's article 'The time to punish and the problem of moral luck'.
9   Williams, *Ethics and the Limits of Responsibility*, and 'Postscript' in Statman (ed.), *Moral Luck*.
10 See, for example, Pamela Salsberry, 'Caring, virtue theory, and a foundation for nursing ethics'; Patricia Benner, 'A dialogue between virtue

ethics and care ethics'; Stan van Hooft, 'Acting from the virtue of caring in nursing'; Edmund D. Pellegrino, 'Toward a virtue-based normative ethics for the health professions'; and Daniel A. Putnam, 'Virtue and the practice of modern medicine'. For counter-arguments, see, for example, Robert M. Veatch, 'The danger of virtue', and H. Tristram Engelhardt Jr., 'The crisis of virtue'.

11　Ronald Dworkin, *Sovereign Virtue*, p. 73.

12　White, 'Rational self-sufficiency', p. 140, is the inspiration for this example.

13　Nagel, 'Moral luck', p. 28.

14　Ibid.

15　Alison van Rooy, 'Good news! You may be out of a job: reflections on the past and future 50 years for Northern NGOs', p. 36.

16　Nagel, 'Moral luck', p. 60.

17　Walker, 'Geographies of responsibility', p. 39, citing Joel Feinberg, *Doing and Deserving*.

18　Card, *The Unnatural Lottery*.

19　From Williams, 'A critique of utilitarianism'. Williams advances the example in a discussion of negative responsibility, and further discussion of it has often been in this light (e.g. John Harris, *Violence and Responsibility*, p. 110 ff.) In this chapter I do not intend to deal with negative responsibility (e.g. responsibility for outcomes which one has omitted to prevent), although those questions will recur later, for example in the chapter on distribution of scarce medical resources. Here my concern is with the decision-theoretical question of whether Williams has given us all the possible outcomes. For simplicity's sake, I use Harris's recast version of the example; in the original, Pedro is the captain's helper.

20　Williams, 'Critique', p. 117.

21　Ibid., p. 109.

22　Williams, 'Utilitarianism and moral self-indulgence', p. 43.

23　Ibid., original emphasis.

24　Ibid.

25　Williams, 'Moral Luck', p. 20, attributing the term 'unconditioned' to Kant. Note the consistency of defining chance merely as contingency, rather than as that of whose likelihood nothing can be known. This is also consistent with decision theories, much of whose purpose is to minimize our ignorance about the workings of chance.

26　Nagel, 'Moral luck', p. 35.

27　Ibid., p. 38.

28　Williams, 'Moral luck', p. 29.

29　See, *inter alia*, Tom L. Beauchamp and James F. Childress, *Principles of Biomedical Ethics*; Raanan Gillon, *Philosophical Medical Ethics*; and H. Tristram Engelhardt Jr., *The Foundations of Bioethics*. For critiques of the autonomy-centred view, see, *inter alia*, Daniel Callahan, 'Can the moral commons survive autonomy?'; Thomas Murray, 'Attending to particulars'; Hilde and James Lindemann Nelson, *The Patient in the Family*; and Michael Parker and Donna Dickenson, *The Cambridge Medical Ethics Workbook*, chapter 8, 'Thinking about autonomy and patient choice', pp. 269–311. I use the Kantian notion of substantive autonomy in preference to the Humean notion of formal autonomy, which is less vulnerable to the moral luck paradox but which has also had much less influence in medical ethics. See the discussion on p. 281 of Veikko Launis, 'The concept of personal autonomy', in Parker and Dickenson.

30 See, for example, several of the articles in chapter 1 of Fulford, Dickenson and Murray (eds), *The Blackwell Reader in Healthcare Ethics and Human Values*.

31 Zimmerman, 'Luck and moral responsibility', p. 374.

32 Williams, 'Postscript,' p. 252.

33 Williams, 'Moral luck', p. 36, n. 11.

34 E.g. in *Ethics and the Limits of Philosophy*.

35 Hindsight clearly offers no help with the decision we are facing now, unless it is hindsight about a genuinely similar previous decision. Establishing what is a genuinely similar previous decision is notoriously fraught. At the time of the Vietnam War, it was widely argued that the 'domino' policy which the United States was pursuing in South-East Asia was based on the incorrect assumption that Vietnam was another Sudetenland or Rheinland, and that 'appeasing' America's enemies in Vietnam was the equivalent mistake to Chamberlain's appeasement of Hitler.

36 Williams, 'Moral luck', p. 23.

37 Ibid., p. 25.

38 Ibid.

39 Nagel, 'Moral luck', p. 28, n. 3.

40 Statman's suggestion, *Moral Luck*, p. 21.

41 Williams, 'Moral luck', p. 26.

42 Ibid., p. 27.

43 Lev Nikolaievich Tolstoy, *Anna Karenina*, p. 17.

44 Karenin refuses to grant Anna a divorce, so that the formal marriage persists, but not the marital relationship.

45 Williams, 'Moral luck', p. 26.

46 For a contrasting view from another feminist philosopher, see Claudia Card, *Unnatural Lottery*, p. 37: 'If her husband Alexey Alexandrovitch, her lover Vronsky, some of her former society friends, and sexist social norms were also responsible, that is a separate point. Her responsibility is determinable somewhat independently of others', in terms of the risks of her own choices.'

47 Andre, 'Nagel, Williams and moral luck', p. 206.

48 Margaret Urban Walker (then Coyne), 'Moral luck?' pp. 322–3, cited in Card, *Unnatural Lottery*, p. 38.
49 Taken from Carolyn Faulder, *Whose Body Is It?*, p. 9. In fact the trial was approved by eleven research ethics committees, not one.
50 For a similar argument, see Erich Loewy, 'The uncertainty of certainty in clinical ethics'.
51 Williams, 'Moral luck', p. 38.
52 Nicholas Rescher, 'Moral luck', p. 158.
53 Norvin Richards, 'Luck and desert', pp. 167–8.
54 Margaret Urban Walker, 'Moral luck and the virtues of impure agency'.

Chapter 2   The Fragility of Virtue and the Robust Health of Kantianism

1 This is an extremely rough summary of Williams's further development of his thinking in *Ethics and the Limits of Philosophy*.
2 For example, I have myself criticized Martha Nussbaum's *Women and Human Development* on those grounds, saying: 'Nussbaum needs an account of what it is to be human which overcomes such cultural relativism, but too much rests on rhetorical terms like "dignity," "human" and "flourishing". This becomes clear if we substitute "dog" for "person" and "canine" for "human" in this sentence: "...beneath a certain level of capability, in each area, a person has not been enabled to live in a truly human way" (Nussbaum, p. 74).' (Dickenson, review of Nussbaum's *Women and Human Development*).
3 E.g., Michael Slote, *From Morality to Virtue*, and 'Virtue ethics', in Marcia W. Baron, Philip Pettit and Michael Slote, *Three Methods of Ethics*.
4 Edmund Pellegrino, e.g., in 'Toward a virtue-based normative ethics', takes the view that the health care professions, which can agree on the *telos* of healing, are more fertile grounds for virtue ethics than is any society in general. See also Edmund D. Pellegrino and David Thomasma, *The Virtues in Medical Practice*. For a clear summary of the rise of virtue ethics in bioethics, see Justin Oakley, 'A virtue ethics approach'.
5 For an extremely clear analysis of this distinction, see Richard Ashcroft, 'Teaching for patient-centred ethics in medicine'.
6 Daniel Putnam, 'Virtue and the practice of modern medicine'.
7 For example, English law on medical negligence sets the standard of negligence as 'practice accepted as proper by a responsible body of medical men skilled in that particular act' (Bolam *v.* Friern Hospital Management Committee [1957] 1 W.L.R. 582, at 586). The merely non-negligent practitioner is of course not the same as the fully virtuous

practitioner, but, insofar as not being negligent is a bottom line under virtue, it can be seen that what is regarded as good practice can shift in accordance with what comes to be accepted over time. See also Margaret Brazier and Jose Miola, 'Bye-bye *Bolam*: a medical litigation revolution?'.

8 Among many entries in a large literature, see, for example, Pamela Salsberry, 'Caring, virtue theory, and a foundation for nursing ethics'; Stan van Hooft, 'Acting from the virtue of caring in nursing'; David Robertson, 'Ethical theory, ethnography, and differences between doctors and nurses in approaches to patient care'; Linda Hanford, 'Nursing and the concept of care: an appraisal of Noddings's theory'; Peter Allmark, 'Can there be an ethics of care?', and Ann Bradshaw, 'Yes! There is an ethics of care: an answer for Peter Allmark'. I have put 'caring' in inverted commas because it is not entirely clear to me that the word describes a virtue rather than an action. If there is a virtue, it must lie in being a 'caring' person, but exactly what that means is also unclear to me. Van Hooft claims that caring is itself a virtue, which in turn dictates other virtues such as sensitivity and concern. This seems to make 'caring' into an umbrella concept and to rob it of precise meaning.

9 Walker, 'Moral luck and the virtues of impure agency', p. 240.

10 Quoted in Steven Morris, Helen Carter and Andrew Osborn, 'Damning verdict on doctor who practised deception', *The Guardian*, 31 January 2001, section 1, p. 4.

11 Walker, 'Moral luck and the virtues of impure agency', p. 240.

12 Ibid., p. 241.

13 Charles Taylor, *Sources of the Self*, p. 3.

14 For a fuller elaboration of this view, see, in addition to Walker, John Mackie, *Ethics*; Iris Murdoch, *The Sovereignty of Good*; and John McDowell, 'Virtue and reason'.

15 Walker, 'Moral luck and the virtues of impure agency', p. 244.

16 See, for example, Pellegrino, 'Toward a virtue-based normative ethics', and Candace Gauthier, 'Teaching the virtues'.

17 See, for Greece, Alasdair MacIntyre, *After Virtue*; for nineteenth-century America, Donna Dickenson, *Margaret Fuller: Writing a Woman's Life*.

18 Robert Veatch, 'The danger of virtue'. A similar argument is made by Erich Loewy in 'Developing habits and knowing what habits to develop'. Robert Louden makes the slightly different point that the virtue approach tells us too little about what to do in the concrete situation facing us here and now (Louden, 'On some vices of virtue ethics', p. 229).

19 Walker, 'Moral luck and the virtues of impure agency', p. 243.

20 See, for example, Oakley, 'A virtue ethics approach', p. 299; Rosalind Hursthouse, 'Normative virtue ethics', *passim*.

21   Nussbaum, *The Fragility of Goodness*, p. 3. See also note 2, for my own criticism that Nussbaum relies too heavily on the rhetorical freight of 'human'.
22   Ibid., p. 3.
23   Ibid., p. 2, original emphasis.
24   Nicholas P. White, in his review 'Rational self-sufficiency and Greek ethics', has queried whether this link between the vulnerability and the value of human endeavour was actually of much concern to the Greeks, suggesting that Nussbaum's thought shows more influence from Bernard Williams in this respect.
25   This is a startling claim, given the dominance of ethical consequential-ism in much Anglo-American moral philosophy. Consequentialism's position in relation to moral luck will be examined in chapter 3.
26   Williams, 'Ethical consistency', p. 173.
27   Nussbaum, *Fragility of Goodness*, p. 25.
28   Ibid., p. 36.
29   Ibid., p. 50.
30   MacIntyre, *After Virtue*, p. 3.
31   Nussbaum, *Fragility of Goodness*, p. 5.
32   Immanuel Kant, *Lectures on Ethics*, p. 132 ('Conscience').
33   Nussbaum, *Fragility of Goodness*, p. 63, discussing Antigone.
34   Nagel, *The View from Nowhere*, p. 195ff. Further permutations are available if we introduce a third element, the rational, as Nagel illus-trates.
35   See, for example, Moira Gatens, *Feminism and Philosophy*; Joan Cocks, *The Oppositional Imagination*; and Nancy C. M. Hartsock, *Money, Sex and Power: toward a feminist historical materialism*, especially chapter 10 and appendix 2.
36   Donna Dickenson, *Property, Women and Politics*, p. 42ff.
37   Nagel, *View from Nowhere*, p. 194.
38   Ibid., p. 196.
39   Susan Moller Okin, 'John Rawls', p. 182.
40   Dickenson, *Property, Women and Politics*, p. 103.
41   Seyla Benhabib, 'On Hegel, Women and Irony', p. 135.
42   However, although Rawls has incorporated some feminist criticisms into the revised version of *A Theory of Justice*, he remains insensitive to women's rights to education and employment in his *The Law of Peoples*.
43   White, 'Rational self-sufficiency', p. 140.
44   Beck, preface to Kant, *Lectures on Ethics*, p. xii.
45   Blum, *Friendship, Altruism and Morality*, p. 31ff.
46   White, 'Rational self-sufficiency', p. 143.
47   Nagel, 'Moral luck', p. 24.
48   Nussbaum, *Fragility of Goodness*, p. 399.

49 Ibid., n. 7, p. 52.
50 Roger Scruton, *Kant*, pp. 72–3.
51 Kant, *The Metaphysics of Morals*, section 221, p. 21, original emphasis.
52 Kant, *Critique of Practical Reason*, preface, p. 4, n. 1.
53 Scruton, *Kant*, p. 64, original emphasis.
54 Kant, *Lectures*, 'Responsibilities for consequences of actions', p. 59.
55 Ibid., p. 60.
56 Scruton, *Kant*, p. 66.
57 Kant, *Lectures*, p. 60, original emphasis.
58 Ibid., p. 62.
59 For a fuller discussion of the disciplinary jurisdiction of the General Medical Council and the United Kingdom Central Council for Nursing, Health Visiting and Midwifery, see Jonathan Montgomery, *Health Care Law*, p. 145ff.
60 Kant, *Critique of Practical Reason*, p. 8, n. 5.
61 Kant, *Metaphysics of Morals*, part 2, section 213, p. 11.
62 Ibid., section 220, p. 19.
63 Kant, *Fundamental Principles of the Metaphysic of Morals*, p. 26, emphasis added. Page references are to those bracketed in the text, from the German edition edited by Rosencranz and Schubert in 1838.
64 Cited in Blum, *Friendship, Altruism and Morality*, p. 26.
65 Kant, *Fundamental Principles*, p. 12.
66 Kant, *Lectures*, p. 65.

Chapter 3 Utilitarianism and Luck in Outcomes

1 For an assessment of the value of this literature and of its technological bent, see Robert Nozick, *The Nature of Rationality*.
2 G. E. Moore, *Ethics*; Bertrand Russell, *Philosophical Essays*; C. D. Broad, 'The doctrine of consequences in ethics'.
3 As Broad phrases Russell's argument, in 'The doctrine of consequences', p. 27.
4 Broad, 'The doctrine of consequences', p. 29.
5 Ibid., p. 35.
6 Ibid., p. 26.
7 A. N. Prior, 'The consequences of actions'.
8 Ibid., p. 96.
9 Richard Brandt, *A Theory of the Good and the Right*, p. 153.
10 On this point, see Reichenbach, 'On the justification of induction', quoted in G. H. von Wright, *The Logical Problem of Induction*, p. 108n: 'Belief can be the *motive* of action, but belief as such can never *justify* an action; only a *justified* belief can do that.' See also Brandt, *Good and Right*, p. 71.

11   See, for example, Jonathan Glover, *Causing Death and Saving Lives*, chapter 6, 'Ends and means: double effect'.
12   For example, see the introduction by Helga Kuhse and Peter Singer to their edited volume *Bioethics: an anthology*.
13   Broad, 'The doctrine of consequences', p. 28.
14   Calculated, for the USA in 1975, from table 2 in S. Liechtenstein et al., 'Judged frequency of lethal events'.
15   Taken from Charles Nesson, 'Reasonable doubt and permissible inference'.
16   L. Jonathan Cohen, *The Probable and the Provable*, p. 120.
17   Robert Nozick, *The Nature of Rationality*, p. 91, in discussing another paradox of probability, Henry Kyburg's 'lottery paradox'. The essence of the lottery paradox is that it is irrational of me to believe that any ticket in a lottery will win, because the probability of each ticket's winning is minuscule, and yet it is also irrational of me to believe that no ticket will win. (From Henry Kyburg Jr., *Probability and the Logic of Rational Belief*, pp. 196–9.) There are parallels here to Nesson's case, but the difference is that no *a priori* ethical or legal principle is involved.
18   Nozick, *The Nature of Rationality*, p. 35.
19   Ibid., p. 36.
20   Ibid., p. 139.
21   Ibid., especially chapter 4.
22   Kuhse and Singer, 'Introduction', in *Bioethics*, p. 3.
23   J. J. C. Smart, in Smart and Williams, *Utilitarianism: for and against*, pp. 40–1.
24   Jeremy Bentham, *Pauper Management Improved*, quoted in Nussbaum, *Fragility of Goodness*, p. 89.
25   Bernard Williams, 'Moral luck', p. 25.
26   E.g., Archie Cochrane, *Effectiveness and Efficiency*.
27   Williams, 'Moral luck', p. 31.
28   Ibid., p. 25.
29   Letter from Dr Tony Fogarty, *The Guardian*, 23 July 2001, p. 19.

Chapter 4   Risk and Consent

1   In the leading English case on consent, *Sidaway* v. *Board of Governors of Bethlem Hospital*, it was held, by Lord Justice Dunn in the Court of Appeal judgment, that 'informed consent is no part of English law'. It is the 'informed' part that is most relevant. Consent is required to avoid an action for battery, but the American doctrine of 'informed' consent is arguably a different matter. For a view that the requirements of consent are becoming more stringent, see Margaret Brazier and Jose Miola, 'Bye-bye *Bolam*'; see also Bolitho *v.* City and Hackney Health Authority (1998).

2   I refer here to the competent adult patient; for a further discussion of incompetent adult patients, and of potentially competent young people under eighteen, see chapter 8.

3   Schloendorff *v.* Society of NY Hospitals (1914).

4   Natanson *v.* Kline (1960), quoted in Carolyn Faulder, *Whose Body Is It?*, p. 14.

5   Canterbury *v.* Spence (1972).

6   State of Massachusetts statute, 1979, quoted in Faulder, *Whose Body Is It?*, p. 14.

7   M. D. Kirby, 'Informed consent: what does it mean?'.

8   Bolitho *v.* City and Hackney Health Authority (1998) has been adduced as a sign of a fundamental shift in English law. Brazier and Miola, in 'Bye-bye *Bolam*', agree that *Bolitho*, together with other cases, the role of the National Institute of Clinical Excellence in issuing guidelines for good practice, and proposals by the Law Commission and the Department of Health, all signal a shift away from unfettered medical power, although there are few risks to doctors' professional integrity and independence (p. 86).

9   Here I am deliberately oversimplifying the jurisprudence for the sake of developing a philosophically interesting contrast.

10 Lord Scarman's minority opinion in *Sidaway* does adopt the 'prudent patient' standard, in relation to the doctor's duty to disclose information about the risks of proposed treatment.

11 I owe this suggestion to Alan Ryan.

12 Bolam *v.* Friern Hospital Management Committee (1957).

13 Ibid., at 587.

14 Brazier and Miola, 'Bye-bye *Bolam*', p. 90.

15 Again making a partial exception for Lord Scarman's dissent, in which he remarked that *Bolam*, as a negligence case, was an inappropriate standard by which to judge the very different issues of consent in *Sidaway*.

16 *Bolitho*, at 392, cited in Brazier and Miola, 'Bye-bye *Bolam*', p. 105.

17 *Bolitho*, n. 3 at 243, cited in ibid., p. 108.

18 Smith *v.* Tunbridge Wells Health Authority (1994).

19 Pearce *v.* United Bristol Healthcare NHS Trust (1999).

20 Ibid., at 59, cited in Brazier and Miola, 'Bye-bye *Bolam?*', p. 109, emphasis added.

21 See, for example, chapter 18, 'Consent', in Raanan Gillon, *Philosophical Medical Ethics*.

22 Diana Brahams, 'To be perfectly frank'.

23 Reported in D. Oken, 'What to tell cancer patients'.

24 See, for the UK, Clive Seale and A. Cartwright, *The Year before Death*, and Clive Seale, 'Demographic change and the experience of dying'; for the USA, D. H. Novack et al., 'Changes in physicians' attitudes toward

telling the cancer patient'. Novack and his colleagues found that 98 per cent of physicians questioned had a policy of telling cancer patients their diagnosis. It is at least arguable, however, that transformations in American doctors' beliefs are a reflection rather than a cause of changes in American law.

25 Eric Wilkes, *A Sourcebook in Terminal Care*, summarized in Alan G. Johnson, *Pathways in Medical Ethics*, p. 122, fig. 14.9.

26 See, for example, Robert M. Veatch and Sara T. Fry, *Case Studies in Nursing Ethics*, p. 124; Gwen Adshead and Donna Dickenson, 'Why do doctors and nurses disagree?'; and Basiro Davey, 'The nurse's dilemma: truth-telling or big white lies?'.

27 Alastair Campbell, *Moderated Love*, chapters 2 and 3.

28 Gill Crabbe, 'The ultimate test'.

29 This was the conclusion of the working party of the UK Institute of Medical Ethics (see Kenneth M. Boyd, 'HIV infection: ethics of anonymised testing') as well as of the noted epidemiologist Sir Richard Doll, who was widely reported as saying that no one was harmed by screening, whereas much general benefit to the population could thus be obtained.

30 For arguments against this policy, see Paquita de Zuleuta, 'The ethics of anonymised HIV testing of pregnant women: a reappraisal', and 'HIV in pregnancy'.

31 This example is discussed at greater length in chapter 6.

32 For further discussion of the limitations of EBM, see Tony Hope, 'Editorial'; Donna Dickenson and Paolo Viners, 'Evidence-based medicine and quality of care'; Donna Dickenson, 'Can medical criteria settle priority-setting debates?'; and S. Harrison, 'The politics of evidence-based medicine'.

33 Bernard Williams, 'The self and the future' and 'Persons, character and morality'.

34 Much of this account is drawn from David McCarthy, 'Rights, explanations and risks'.

35 Judith Jarvis Thomson, *The Realm of Rights* and *Rights, Restitution and Risk*.

36 Robert Nozick, *Anarchy, State and Utopia*.

37 For the opposite argument, see Donna Dickenson, 'The right to know and the right to privacy'.

38 See J. K. Mason, 'The legal aspects and implications of risk assessment'.

39 John Hinton, *Dying*, p. 81: 'Anxiety seems about equally common in those who recognize that their lives may be about to end and those who apparently do not.'

40 See, for example, Clough, 'The validation of meaning'; Wallace, 'Informed consent in elective surgery'; and Weinman, 'Providing written information for patients'.

41 Reported in Weinman, 'Providing written information for patients'.
42 Ibid.
43 For a rather extreme version of this argument, see Mark S. Komrad, 'A defence of medical paternalism', and Richard Sherlock's untitled contribution to the symposium on consent, competence and electro-convulsive therapy in the *Journal of Medical Ethics*. A milder version of the argument can be found in John Kleinig, *Ethical Issues in Psychosurgery*, p. 19.
44 For further discussion of one such abuse, in the case of Mr L, a man with learning difficulties and autism, see Ajit Shah and Donna Dickenson, 'The *Bournewood* case'; Ajit Shah and Donna Dickenson, 'The capacity to make decisions in dementia', and Donna Dickenson and Ajit Shah, 'The *Bournewood* judgement: a way forward?'.
45 For a list of cases and discussion of the legal and clinical issues, see Wendy Savage, 'Caesarean section – who chooses?'
46 Case 4 in Tom L. Beauchamp and James F. Childress, *Principles of Biomedical Ethics*, 2nd edn, pp. 228–9.
47 I am thinking particularly of the Caroline Spear case (1992), discussed by Savage in 'Caesarean section – who chooses?'
48 Case 7 in Tom L. Beauchamp and James F. Childress, *Principles of Biomedical Ethics*, 2nd edn, p. 291.
49 The words of a nurse who attended a day seminar I ran on ethical and professional issues for nursing staff at the John Radcliffe Hospital, Oxford, in March 1987.
50 As suggested by Alan Donagan in 'Informed consent in theory and experimentation'.
51 Robert Buckman, *I Don't Know What to Say*, p. 29.
52 Salgo *v.* Leland Stanford Jr. University Board of Trustees (1957).
53 E.g., by James Fries and Elizabeth Loftus in their correspondence with Ruth Barcan Marcus, Bruce Kuklick and Saevan Bercovich in *Science* (1979).
54 Ruth Faden et al., 'Disclosure of information to patients in medical care'.
55 *Which?* magazine survey by Consumers' Association, 7 February 1991.
56 Richard Brandt, *Good and Right*, p. 10.
57 Ibid., p. 11.
58 George Robinson and Avram Merar, 'Informed consent: recall by patients,' p. 182 ff.
59 Ibid., p. 184.
60 For an example of this fallacious reasoning, see Franz J. Ingelfinger, 'Informed (but uneducated) consent'.
61 Alastair Campbell and Roger Higgs, *In That Case*, p. 28.
62 Sard *v.* Hardy (1977).
63 Canterbury *v.* Spence (1972), emphasis added. See also Wilkinson *v.* Vesey (1972) and Cobbs *v.* Grant (1972).

64   Loren Roth, Alan Meisel and Charles Lidz, 'Tests of competency to consent'.
65   Re W (1992).
66   Re C (1994).
67   Lake *v.* Cameron ([1967] 267 F.Supp. 155).

Chapter 5   Death and Dying

1   British Medical Association, *Children's Consent to Medical Treatment.* The pioneer in this field was probably Priscilla Alderson, particularly her books *Choosing for Children* and *Children's Consent to Surgery.* For a review of the literature, see Donna Dickenson, 'Consent in children'.
2   Royal College of Paediatrics and Child Health, *Report of the Ethics Advisory Committee.*
3   Some of this research is surveyed in Donna Dickenson and David Jones, 'True wishes', and in Donna Dickenson, 'Consent in children'.
4   Airedale NHS Trust *v.* Bland ([1993] 1 All ER 821).
5   Ibid., at p. 859.
6   Keith Andrews et al., 'Misdiagnosis of the vegetative state'.
7   E.g., Frenchay NHS Trust *v.* S ([1994] 2 All ER 403).
8   Cruzan *v.* Director, Missouri Department of Health (1990).
9   Interviewed in BBC1's 'Heart of the Matter', 3 March 1991.
10   Sheila McLean, 'Is there a legal threat to medicine?', p. 3.
11   Dickenson, *Moral Luck in Medical Ethics and Practical Politics*, p. 127.
12   Ibid.
13   For further discussion of these issues, see Gillian Craig, 'On withholding nutrition and hydration', and the replies by Ashby and Stoffell and R. J. Dunlop et al.
14   D. P. T. Price, 'Organ transplant initiatives'.
15   Per Lord Musthill, at p. 894.
16   F. *v.* West Berkshire Health Authority, at 566, per Lord Goff.
17   E.g., Re E (1993).
18   For a more complete discussion of this point, see Eve Gerrard, 'Palliative care and the ethics of resource allocation'. Resource allocation and moral luck are discussed in chapter 6 of the present book.
19   Discussed by Alex J. London and Lori P. Knowles in 'The Maltese conjoined twins' and the letter of reply by Pierre Mallia.
20   Washington et al. *v.* Glucksberg and Vacco *v.* Quill.
21   For an example of this style of argument, see Hazel Curry, 'A dignified death'.
22   For further discussion of this point, see Dworkin, *Sovereign Virtue*, p. 470.

23 It is rather surprising that Dworkin does not himself make this connection; he favours legalization of assisted suicide and accepts the Fourteenth Amendment arguments raised in the Washington and New York circuit court of appeals cases. See *Sovereign Virtue*, chapter 14, 'Sex, death and the courts'.

24 The applicability of the traditional Catholic doctrine of double effect to such cases in English law was established in the 1997 case of Annie Lindsell, who suffered from motor neurone disease. It was held that doctors already possessed the power to prescribe pain-relieving medication for Miss Lindsell that might have the side effect of hastening her death, although the court stopped short of ruling that her mental distress could also be relieved in such fashion.

25 Airedale NHS Trust *v*. Bland, at p. 866.

26 Savulescu and Dickenson, 'The time frame of preferences'.

27 Law Commission, *Mentally Incapacitated Adults and Decision-Making* (Consultation Paper no. 129) and *Mental Incapacity* (Report no. 231); Lord Chancellor's Department, *Who Decides?* and *Making Decisions*.

28 Re C (1994), Re T (1992).

29 Lord Chancellor's Department, *Making Decisions*, paragraph 19, p. 4.

30 Joan M. Teno et al., 'Do formal advance directives affect resuscitation decisions?'

31 Christopher Ryan, 'Betting your life,' p. 291.

32 Daniel Callahan, *The Troubled Dream of Life*, especially chapter 1.

33 Derek Parfit, *Reasons and Persons*, p. 148ff.

34 C. Owen et al., 'Suicide and euthanasia', cited in Ryan, p. 293.

35 M. Danis et al., 'Stability of choices about life-sustaining treatments', cited in Ryan, p. 293.

36 P. Alleback et al., 'Increased suicide risk in cancer patients', cited in Ryan, p. 294.

37 Other studies, not cited by Ryan, do confirm that people adapt to conditions such as paraplegia which they might once have thought 'worse than death'. See Kahneman and Varey, 'Notes on the psychology of utility'; Argyle, *The Psychology of Happiness*; Taylor, *Positive Illusions*; Silver and Wortman, 'Coping with undesirable life events'; and Vaillant, *Adaptation to Life*.

38 *Re C* upheld this right in the case of a schizophrenic with delusions felt by his clinicians to compromise his ability to refuse treatment. See also the statement by Lord Templeman in *Sidaway* that 'The patient is entitled to reject [medical] advice for reasons which are rational, or irrational, or for no reason.'

39 E.g., Tony Hope, 'Advance directives', and the concerns expressed by some respondents to the Lord Chancellor's Department consultation document *Who Decides?*, as summarized in paragraph 14 of *Making Decisions* (p. 3).

40 Joanne Lynn, 'Why I don't have a living will'.
41 Margaret Urban Walker, 'Geographies of responsibility', p. 39, citing Joel Feinberg, *Doing and Deserving*.
42 For a discussion of contract as involving recognition of agency, see Donna Dickenson, *Property, Women and Politics*, chapter 4. To the extent that this is true, and that advance directives represent a form of contract, there are agency-enhancing arguments for their recognition.
43 Dickenson and Jones, 'True wishes'.
44 Robert Graves, *The Greek Myths*, p. 361.
45 Savulescu and Dickenson, 'The time frame of preferences', pp. 232–3.
46 Ibid., p. 233.
47 Ibid., pp. 234–5.

Chapter 6 Moral Luck and the Allocation of Health-Care Resources

1 Guido Calabresi and Philip Bobbitt, *Tragic Choices*.
2 Calabresi and Bobbitt (p. 19) likewise distinguish between first- and second-order determinations.
3 Dickenson, 'Is efficiency ethical?', p. 237.
4 R. *v.* Cambridge Health Authority, ex parte B (1995). Child B, later identified as Jaymee Bowen, was acutely ill with leukaemia. Her health authority refused to fund an 'experimental' treatment, on advice from her clinician that she had only six to eight weeks to live and that further treatment was inappropriate. Her father went to court to compel the authority to pay for the treatment; although he succeeded in the High Court, the Court of Appeal ruled against him. The money was later provided by a private donor, and the treatment given, but Jaymee died a few months thereafter.
5 Sanders and Dukeminier, 'Medical advance and legal lag', p. 368.
6 Robert Veatch, *Death, Dying and the Biological Revolution*, pp. 208–9.
7 Calabresi and Bobbitt, *Tragic Choices*, p. 184.
8 Since Calabresi and Bobbitt published *Tragic Choices* in 1978, a more evidence-based system has come to the fore in Italy with the establishment of the Italian Cochrane Centre. (See Paolo Vineis, 'Italy country report'.) The usefulness of the Italian model is now not so much as an up-to-date description of actual practice as an alternative conceptual model stressing equality above clinical criteria.
9 Calabresi and Bobbitt, *Tragic Choices*, p. 182.
10 John Rawls, *A Theory of Justice*.
11 Summarized in footnote 90 to p. 182 of Calabresi and Bobbitt, *Tragic Choices*.
12 Calabresi and Bobbitt, *Tragic Choices*, footnote 93 to p. 183.

13 US *v.* Holmes, cited in James Childress, 'Who shall live when not all can live?', p. 642.

14 In my article 'Are medical ethicists out of touch?', I argue that the prevailing slant among clinicians and in the law is deontological, as against the consequentialist domination of much medical ethics.

15 Veatch and Fry, *Case Studies in Nursing Ethics*, case 23, 'Allocating nursing time according to benefit', p. 84. In addition to my discussion of this case in the first edition of this book, another version appears in my article 'Nurse time as a scarce health care resource'.

16 Robert Buckman, *I Don't Know What to Say*, chapter 5, 'Facing the threat', p. 23ff.

17 Thomas Nagel, *The View from Nowhere*, p. 35.

18 For a further discussion of mental capacity in suicidal patients, see Dickenson and Fulford, *In Two Minds*, case 3, Martin McKendrick.

19 In interviewing nurses on a coronary care unit, David Field found that there was surprisingly little sense of failure when a patient died, so long as the nurses were sure that they had done everything possible to stave off the death. See Field, *Nursing the Dying*, p. 78. A similar finding was reported by Glaser and Strauss in their *Awareness of Dying*.

20 Paul Freund, 'Introduction', p. 13.

21 Neil Duxbury, *Random Justice*.

22 Archie Cochrane, *Effectiveness and Efficiency*.

23 Paolo Vineis, *The Tension between Ethics and Evidence-Based Medicine*.

24 Reidar Lie, commentary at Evibase workshop, Maastricht, 2 February 2001.

25 Tony Hope, 'Editorial: evidence-based medicine and ethics'; Donna Dickenson, 'Can medical criteria settle priority-setting debates?'.

26 Herve Allain, 'New drug therapies: how far can we stretch ethics?'.

27 J. A. Kaasenbrood, 'Evidence based medicine en de dagelijkse psychiatrische praktijk'.

28 M. Berg, 'Problemen en potenties van het protocol, de voorwaarden om protocollen positief in te zetten' and *Rationalizing Medical Work: decision support techniques and medical practices*.

29 A. Stoop, M. Berg, and G. J. Dinant, 'Tussen afwijken en afwijzen van richtlijnen'.

30 S. Harrison, 'The politics of evidence-based medicine in the United Kingdom'.

31 Dickenson, 'Can medical criteria settle priority-setting debates?' and 'Is efficiency ethical?'.

32 Hope, 'Editorial: evidence-based medicine and ethics'.

33 Martin Walker, 'Luck of the draw for MS drug'. Proposals for some form of randomization in allocating scarce health resources can also be found in Winslow, *Triage and Justice*; Outka, 'Social justice and equal

access to health care'; and Green, 'Health care and justice in contract theory perspective'.

34   John Harris, 'QALYfying the value of life'. Of course it is discriminatory in a morally wrong sense only if one believes that we should not necessarily choose younger people above older people. For a defence of this view, see A. B. Shaw, 'In defence of ageism'. See also Daniel Callahan, *Setting Limits*, and Margaret Battin, 'Age rationing and the just distribution of health care'.

35   John Harris, *The Value of Life*, p. 89.

36   Robert Veatch, *Death, Dying and the Biological Revolution*, pp. 204–5.

37   Nancy Jecker, 'Caring for "socially undesirable" patients'.

38   Beauchamp and Childress, *Principles of Biomedical Ethics*, 4th edn, p. 385. The AMA Council on Ethical and Judicial Affairs also believes that: 'Social worth considerations would destroy the public confidence in physicians' abilities to place patients' interests above broad social utility.' ('Ethical Considerations in the Allocation of Organs and Other Scarce Medical Resources among Patients', *Archives of Internal Medicine*, 155 (1995), 29–40, at p. 32.)

39   Harris, *Value of Life*, p. 106.

40   Jonathan Glover, *Causing Death and Saving Lives*, p. 222.

41   Anna Coote and Beatrix Campbell, *Sweet Freedom*, p. 89.

42   Ibid., pp. 63–7, 164, 261–2.

43   Harris often conflates misfortune and injustice, I feel, as in his claim that it is somehow unjust not to live to the statistical norm of seventy (*Value of Life*, p. 93).

Chapter 7   Reproductive Ethics: What Risks Can Women be Asked to Bear?

1   See Susan Dodds and Kathleen Jones, 'Surrogacy and autonomy', and the response by Justin Oakley, 'Altruistic surrogacy'.

2   In the UK the Human Organ Transplant Act 1989 prohibits commercial trading in kidneys and other organs. Sixteen other European countries have similar legislation, and the European Convention on Human Rights bans international trade in organs. In the United States the Transplantation of Human Organs Act 1984 makes it illegal to 'knowingly acquire, receive or otherwise transfer any human organ for valuable consideration for use in human transplantation if the transfer affects interstate commerce.' India, which was widely condemned for allowing illicit trade in human organs to flourish, has now taken steps to stop the trade with its Transplantation of Human Organs Act (1992). A summary of this legislation can be found on p. 199 of the British Medical Association handbook *The Medical Profession and Human*

Rights. The BMA has considered and rejected the argument that selling a kidney at least allows a needy person to live, and that the choice should be up to those living in poverty: 'The BMA does not believe that condoning such exploitative relationships is an appropriate way to tackle the effects of poverty' (p. 200).

3 Robert G. Lee and Derek Morgan, *Human Fertilisation and Embry-ology*, p. 212, n. 19.

4 Ibid.

5 Jamie Wilson and Julian Borger, 'Surrogate twins find new parents'.

6 Advice from an anonymous referee for Polity.

7 Helena Ragone, in *Surrogate Motherhood*, p. 75, confirms that many 'surrogates' do indeed feel this way.

8 For further discussion of the medical and ethical issues involved in 'reduction' or, more properly, pregnancy preservation with termination of one or more foetuses, see Mary B. Mahowald, 'The fewer the better?'.

9 Wendy Savage, 'Caesarean section', p. 260. The death rate for elective Caesareans, at 14.8 per 100,000, still represents a greatly increased risk over vaginal delivery.

10 Helena Ragone, *Surrogate Motherhood*, p. 62.

11 Ibid., p. 67. Ragone believes that many 'surrogates' welcome the shift in the balance of power with their husbands, not only in sexual matters but more generally, while at the same time maintaining the semblance of traditional gender roles by reiterating their desire to 'give the gift of life'.

12 *Daily Telegraph*, 23 February 1994, cited in Lee and Morgan, *Human Fertilisation and Embryology*, p. 193.

13 I presume that the couple have such rights because US law is generally more slanted towards genetic parenthood (e.g., Anna J. *v.* Mark C., and *In the Matter of Baby M*, where a commissioning father was given custody of a child whom the surrogate mother wished to keep, on the grounds that the child was already his by virtue of his genetic input. (See also n. 19, p. 205, of my *Property, Women and Politics.*) The 'surrogate' and her husband are regarded as legal parents of the child in only a very small minority of US states (Arizona, North Dakota and Utah, at the time Helena Ragone performed her research on 'surrogacy' in 1994: see Ragone, *Surrogate Motherhood*, p. 49). In California law the genetic parents appear to be the legal parents; indeed, that may be why they wanted the 'surrogate' to undergo IVF, so as to fend off any countervailing claim from her based on her own genetic input. In English law it would be clear, I think, that the birth mother has sole parental responsibility, unless the genetic father filed for parental responsibility under the provisions of the Children Act 1989, as any father can do who is not married to the child's mother at the time of birth. Whether such an action would succeed is doubtful, I think, in that the genetic father is married to someone else, and in that the 'surrogate's' husband is already

the legal father. A married commissioning couple can file under the 'parental order' section (s30) of the Human Fertilisation and Embryology Act 1990, although there have been at least two cases in which commissioning fathers whose wives have died have been unable to establish parental responsibility in this manner, because only married couples can apply under s30 (Lee and Morgan, *Human Fertilisation and Embryology*, p. 201).

14   Catherine Bennett, 'The baby incubators'.

15   Warnock Report, para 8.2, cited in Lee and Morgan, *Human Fertilisation and Embryology*, p. 198.

16   John Harris, *Clones, Genes and Immortality*, p. 145ff.

17   E.g., Ruth Macklin, 'Is there anything wrong with surrogate motherhood?'; Lori B. Andrews, 'Surrogate motherhood: the challenge for feminists'. Rosemarie Tong formerly advocated that commercial 'surrogacy' should be banned, but that non-commercial 'surrogacy' should be allowed and its procedures amalgamated with those of adoption. She now argues that all forms of gestational motherhood can be dealt with under modified adoption laws. See Rosemarie Tong, 'The overdue death of a feminist chameleon' for the earlier position, and 'Feminist perspectives and gestational motherhood' for the later one.

18   In some states – including California, as of 1994, when Helena Ragone conducted her 'surrogate' interviews there – commercial 'surrogacy' is banned, as is the involvement of third parties (for-profit agencies).

19   Joan Mahoney, 'Adoption as a feminist alternative to reproductive technology' and 'An essay on surrogacy and feminist thought'.

20   In 1991 the first frozen embryo was shipped from England and implanted into the womb of an American 'surrogate' (Helena Ragone, *Surrogate Motherhood*, p. 6).

21   A similar argument is made by Lori Andrews in 'Alternative modes of reproduction'.

22   Anna J. *v.* Mark C. (1991). See also the discussion by Joan Callahan, 'Reconsidering parenthood: introduction', pp. 20–1: 'When Anna Johnson decided she wanted to keep the child, it was held by the court that the genetic progenitors were the legal parents, and that she had no legal claim whatever to parenthood of the child.' On appeal (Johnson *v.* Calvert, 1993) the judgment concerning the primacy of genetic parenthood was confirmed, but not on the grounds of the enforceability of the contract (Lee and Morgan, *Human Fertilisation and Embryology*, p. 214, n. 48).

23   For a more extended, Lockean argument in favour of women's ownership of their property in labour and childbirth, see chapter 3 of my *Property, Women and Politics*.

24   Even by Margaret Brazier, chair of the Brazier Committee, who wrote elsewhere: 'If an infertile couple can buy an egg, and *rent a womb*, why should they not buy the finished product?' (Brazier, 'Can you buy

children?', p. 345, cited in Lee and Morgan, *Human Fertilisation and Embryology*, p. 206). Although Brazier goes on to argue that they should not buy the product, my point here is that she too uses the incorrect language of 'renting a womb', which ignores what women do in the labour of childbirth.

25 Judge Johnson in Johnson *v.* Calvert, cited in Lee and Morgan, *Human Fertilisation and Embryology*, p. 202.
26 Carole Pateman, *The Sexual Contract*, pp. 212–13.
27 Some jurisdictions, including California, have drafted legislation to protect 'surrogate' mothers against such risks as the death of one or both contracting parents or the parents' refusal to take custody of a baby with birth defects. See Ragone, *Surrogate Motherhood*, p. 48.
28 For example, Mahoney, 'Adoption as a feminist alternative'.
29 Helena Ragone, *Surrogate Motherhood*. See also Philip Parker, 'Motivation of surrogate mothers: initial findings'. Parker's findings differ from Ragone's in identifying a greater number of 'surrogates' who acknowledged that they were trying to assuage their guilt in having had an abortion or putting a child up for adoption (Ragone, *Surrogate Motherhood*, p. 62).
30 See the sample advertisements in Ragone, *Surrogate Motherhood*, pp. 30–1.
31 Ragone, *Surrogate Motherhood*, p. 57.
32 An anonymous 'surrogate' interviewed in the *San Diego Union*, 1982, p. D-7, cited in Ragone, *Surrogate Motherhood*, p. 41.
33 Ragone, *Surrogate Motherhood*, p. 11.
34 Ibid., p. 44.
35 Ibid., p. 80.
36 Ibid., p. 45.
37 Ibid., p. 55.
38 Elizabeth Anderson, 'Is women's labor a commodity?'. A similar argument is made by Sandra Marshall in 'Whose child is it anyway?', arguing that the 'surrogate's' non-economic motivation itself renders her vulnerable to exploitation.
39 Professor Alastair Campbell, member of the Brazier Committee, personal communication, October 1998.
40 Margaret Brazier, 'Can you buy children?', p. 345, cited in Lee and Morgan, *Human Fertilisation and Embryology*, p. 206.
41 Michael Freeman, 'Does surrogacy have a future after Brazier?', p. 9, n. 61, cited in Lee and Morgan, *Human Fertilisation and Embryology*, p. 206.
42 Warnock Report, para. 8.17.
43 Department of Health, *Surrogacy*, p. 1.
44 Ibid., p. 2.
45 Martha Field, 'Surrogate motherhood', p. 226.

46   British Medical Association, *Changing Conceptions of Motherhood*. Lee and Morgan argue convincingly that the BMA's change of stance represents a shift from 'surrogacy' as social problem to 'surrogacy' as medical solution – the 'medicalization' of 'surrogacy' as one among many possible remedies for infertility. If so, there is all the more reason to resurrect the language of exploitation before the technocratic language of medicalization becomes all-encompassing.

47   Dickenson, *Property, Women and Politics*, chapter 4.

48   Paragraph b, clause 1, cited in John Harris, *Clones, Genes and Immortality*, p. 31.

49   Harris, *Clones, Genes and Immortality*, p. 31.

50   Julian Borger, 'All sides angry at Bush stem cell decision'; R. Alta Charo, 'Bush's stem cell compromise: a few mirrors?'

51   Boston Women's Health Book Collective, 'Statement on human cloning', June 2001.

52   Donna Dickenson, 'Commodification of human tissue'. See also the comment by Ruth Hubbard, a biologist from the Council for Responsible Genetics in the USA, who criticized the Bush compromise because it would leave the private sector unregulated and free to exploit women: 'Women will be paid to produce eggs just for research – and for profit' (cited in Borger, 'All sides angry at Bush stem cell decision'). An honourable exception to the absence of women from consultation and policy documents is the Health Canada working group report (Discussion Group on Embryo Research, *Research on Human Embryos in Canada*), which made women's health a priority.

53   Gina Kolata, 'Researchers find big risk'; Laura Shanner, *Embryonic Stem Cell Research*, p. 31.

54   Laura Shanner, personal communication, 16 August 2001.

55   As detailed in the US case of 'BX', *Hastings Center Report*, 31: 4 (2001), who developed near-fatal ovarian hyperstimulation syndrome as a result of the injection regime. Other more long-term risks include premature menopause, heart disease and stroke.

56   E.g., Mark A. Wilcox, 'Egg sharing: an NHS consultant's view'.

57   Shanner, *Embryonic Stem Cell Research*, p. 26.

58   For example, at the time of writing, a team at the Institute of Reproductive Medicine and Genetic Testing in California was attempting to derive stem cells through parthenogenesis, from egg cells whose chromosome sets are both from the mother. Another team at PPL Therapeutics in Scotland reported injecting an egg's cytoplasm into an ordinary somatic cell and creating something like a stem cell (Gregory Kaebnick, 'Embryonic stem cells without embryos?').

59   James Meek, 'The brain gain'.

60   Judith Jarvis Thomson, 'A defense of abortion'. One exception is Eileen McDonagh: in *Breaking the Abortion Deadlock* she concedes foetal

personality for the sake of argument, developing a thesis in favour of the right to abortion that is based instead on informed consent.
61 E.g., Julian Savulescu, 'Should we clone human beings?', p. 93.
62 For a further discussion of the concept of exploitation, see Harris, *Clones, Genes, and Immortality*, p. 144ff.
63 Donna Dickenson, 'Property and women's alienation from their own reproductive labour', p. 214.
64 Karl Marx, *Grundrisse*.
65 Donna Dickenson, *Property, Women and Politics*, especially chapter 7. For an application of the theoretical position developed in the book to stem cell technologies, see also my more recent articles 'Property and women's alienation from their own reproductive labour' and 'Commodification of human tissue'.
66 For further discussion, see Dickenson, *Property, Women and Politics*, chapter 5.
67 Medical Research Council, *Report . . . to Develop . . . Guidelines*.
68 Margaret Radin, *Contested Commodities*.
69 Mary Mahowald, 'As if there were foetuses without women'.
70 Moore *v.* Regents of the University of California (1990); Richard Gold, *Body Parts*.

Chapter 8 Psychiatry and Risk

1 A. Maden, 'Risk assessment and management in psychiatry'; Donna Dickenson and K. W. M. Fulford, *In Two Minds*, p. 224.
2 Adapted from Dickenson and Fulford, *In Two Minds*, pp. 226–8.
3 L. Reznek, *The Philosophical Defence of Psychiatry*; K. W. M. Fulford, *Moral Theory and Medical Practice*; T. Szasz, *The Myth of Mental Illness*.
4 General Medical Council, *Good Medical Practice*, p. 13.
5 Donna Dickenson, *Moral Luck in Medical Ethics and Practical Politics*, p. 63.
6 See, for example, the essays in Glyn Davis, Barbara Sullivan and Anna Yeatman (eds), *The New Contractualism*.
7 Donna Dickenson, *Property, Women and Politics*, esp. chapter 4.
8 Thomas Nagel, *The View from Nowhere*, p. 120.
9 Ibid., p. 121.
10 See the commentary by Gwen Adshead on the Alan Masterson case in Dickenson and Fulford, *In Two Minds*, p. 235.
11 R. White, P. Carr and N. Lowe, *A Guide to the Children Act 1989*, p. 102. The notion of significant risk is also enshrined in paragraph 3.72 of the Department of Health's 1994 *Draft Arrangements for Inter-Agency Working for the Care and Protection of Severely Mentally Ill People*.

12   Semler *v.* Psychiatric Institute of Washington (1976); Durflinger *v.* Artiles ([1983] P 2d).
13   Bernard Williams, 'Moral luck', p. 256.
14   Catherine Oppenheimer, 'Ethics and psychogeriatrics', p. 369.
15   E.g., *In re Quinlan, In re Jobes.* For the position in English law, see Jonathan Montgomery, *Health Care Law*, p. 229.
16   Lord Chancellor's Department, *Making Decisions.*
17   Re C (1994).
18   Case 7 in Beauchamp and Childress, *Principles of Biomedical Ethics*, 2nd edn, p. 291.
19   Claudia Card, *The Unnatural Lottery: character and moral luck.*
20   K. W. M. Fulford, *Moral Theory and Medical Practice.*
21   Antony Flew, *A Dictionary of Philosophy*, p. 284.
22   J. K. Mason and R. A. McCall Smith, *Law and Medical Ethics*, p. 411.
23   R. A. Duff, *Intention, Agency and Criminal Liability*, p. 39.
24   Re C (1994).
25   Plato, *Protagoras*, 352b.
26   Alfred R. Mele, *Autonomous Agents*, p. 59.
27   Susan Hurley, *Natural Reasons*, p. 159.
28   Donald Davidson, 'Belief and the basis of meaning', p. 153.
29   Hurley, *Natural Reasons*, p. 159.
30   Mele, *Autonomous Agents*, p. 61.
31   Ibid., p. 63.

Chapter 9   Luck, Genetics and Moral Character

1   Dworkin, *Sovereign Virtue*, p. 444.
2   Ibid.
3   Ibid., p. 446.
4   Nuffield Council on Bioethics, 'Consultation on behavioural genetics' (2001), section 6, <www.nuffieldfoundation.org/bioethics>.
5   Dorothy Nelkin and M. Susan Lindee, *The DNA Mystique.*
6   Ruth Chadwick, 'Gene therapy and personal identity'.
7   W. Gilbert, 'A vision of the grail', p. 83, cited in Chadwick, p. 184.
8   Chadwick, 'Gene therapy and personal identity', p. 184.
9   For a further discussion, see Richard Ashcroft, 'Genetic information and "genetic identity"'.
10   Chadwick, 'Gene therapy and personal identity', p. 185.
11   Ibid., p. 186.
12   IHA/WFN, 'Guidelines for the molecular genetics predictive test in Huntington's Disease'. See also Clinical Genetics Society, 'The genetic testing of children', and Advisory Committee on Genetic Testing, *Report on Genetic Testing for Late-Onset Disorders.*

13 IHA/WFN, 'Guidelines'.
14 Gillick *v.* W. Norfolk and Wisbech AHA (1985).
15 D. G. Sherer and N. G. Repucci, 'Adolescents' capacities to provide voluntary informed consent'.
16 Re T (1992).
17 Re E (1993, 1994).
18 Donna Dickenson and David Jones, 'True wishes', p. 300.
19 Before the risk was lessened through the use of synthetically derived growth hormone.
20 For an extended discussion of such ethical questions in a case involving an adult patient with Huntington's Disease, see Michael Parker and Donna Dickenson, *The Cambridge Medical Ethics Workbook*, pp. 41–2, and Donna Dickenson, 'Psychiatry, ethics and genetics'.
21 I have discussed such cases further in Dickenson, 'Can children and young people consent to testing for adult-onset genetic disorders?', and in Dickenson and Fulford, *In Two Minds*, pp. 197–207.
22 For some of the issues in pre-symptomatic testing for cancer, see Donna Dickenson, 'Ethical issues in pre-cancer testing: the parallel with Huntington's Disease'.
23 R. Smith and B. Wynne, *Expert Evidence*; S. Jasanoff, *Science at the Bar.*
24 For a fuller discussion of the relationship between developments in genetics and clinical psychiatry, see Anthony Pelosi and Anthony David, 'Ethical implications of the new genetics for psychiatry'.
25 J. K. Mason and R. A. McCall Smith, *Law and Medical Ethics*, p. 411.
26 Kevin J. Connolly, 'Genetics of behaviour', p. 286.
27 Catharine MacKinnon, *Feminism Unmodified* and *Toward a Feminist Theory of the State*; Donna Dickenson, *Property, Women and Politics*, p. 8.
28 I. Oswald and J. Evans, 'Serious violence while sleep walking'; P. Fenwick, 'Murdering while asleep'; R.A. McCall Smith, 'When going to sleep is a crime'.
29 Bratty *v.* Attorney-General for Northern Ireland (1963, 1961).
30 Nuffield Council on Bioethics, 'Consultation on behavioural genetics, section 6.
31 Mary Mahowald, *Genes, Women, Equality*, p. 249ff.
32 Victor M. Hesselbrock, 'The genetic epidemiology of alcoholism', cited in Mahowald, p. 249.
33 Mary Mahowald, Genes, *Women, Equality*, p. 321.
34 See also Susan Bewley, 'Restricting the freedom of pregnant women'.
35 Quaid et al., 'Issues in genetic testing for susceptibility to alcoholism'; Plomin et al., *Behavioural Genetics*, both cited in Mahowald, p. 249.
36 Mahowald, *Genes, Women, Equality*, p. 253.
37 Ibid., p. 252.
38 Ibid., p. 253.

39   R. *v.* Quick (1973).
40   See also R. *v.* Bailey (1983); G. Maher, 'Automatism and diabetes'; and G. Maher et al., 'Diabetes mellitus and criminal responsibility'.
41   Guido de Wert et al., *Ethics and Genetics Workbook*, p. 81.
42   Claudia Card, *Unnatural Lottery*, p. 4ff.
43   Dickenson, *Property, Women and Politics*, especially chapter 1; Dickenson, 'Property, particularism and moral persons'.
44   Card, *Unnatural Lottery*, p. 32.
45   Kay Redfield Jamison, *Touched with Fire*, pp. 268–9.
46   Mark S. Bauer, 'Bipolar disorders'.
47   Bertelsen, 'A Danish twin study of manic-depressive disorders', cited in Jamison, p. 193. On the link between genetics and bipolar affective disorder, see *inter alia*: Julien Mendlewicz, 'Genetics of depression and mania', and Ming T. Tsuang and Stephen V. Faraone, *The Genetics of Mood Disorders*. See also the essays in Laura Lee Hall, *Genetics and Mental Illness*, and the Nuffield Council report *Mental Disorder and Genetics: the ethical context* (1998).
48   I have deliberately overstated the case here. In English law adults with mental illness still benefit from the presumption of legal capacity (*Re C*, 1994). However, not all mentally ill adults will be found to have decision-making capacity, and I am depicting Gauguin as one of these people. The test laid down in *Re C*, in relation to capacity to make medical decisions, is threefold: ability to understand and retain treatment information, ability to believe that information, and ability to weigh the information up in making an informed decision. (A subsequent case, *Re MB* [1997], omits the belief component.) If Gauguin was severely affected by bipolar affective disorder, his capacity to weigh up information might well have been seriously imperilled.
49   Nuffield Council on Bioethics, *Mental Disorder and Genetics*, para. 1.3.
50   Thomas Bouchard et al., 'Sources of human psychological differences', p. 223, cited in Mary Mahowald, *Genes, Women, Equality*, p. 244.
51   S. A. Mednick et al., 'Genetic influences in criminal convictions', cited in British Medical Association, *Human Genetics*, p. 200.
52   T. F. McNeil, 'Prebirth and postbirth influence,' cited in Jamison, *Touched with Fire*, p. 85.
53   British Medical Association, *Human Genetics*, p. 36.
54   E.g., Card, *Unnatural Lottery*, p. 3: 'The view that acquisition of the virtues depends in part on externals... implies constitutive moral luck [in] the circumstances of our birth and our early childhoods.'
55   Ibid., p. 31.
56   Ibid., p. 19.
57   In a vast literature, see, for example, Carol Gilligan, *In a Different Voice*; Moira Gatens, 'Power, bodies and difference'; and Gill Jaggar, 'Beyond essentialism and construction'.

58 Card, *Unnatural Lottery*, p. 21.
59 Thomas Nagel, *Mortal Questions*, cited in Card, *Unnatural Lottery*, p. 21.
60 Card, *Unnatural Lottery*, p. 21.
61 For a collection of accounts in which survivors of child abuse detail the many ways in which they have overcome their ill-luck, see Caroline Malone et al. (eds), *The Memory Bird*.
62 Nagel, *View from Nowhere*, p. 127.
63 Card, *Unnatural Lottery*, p. 39.
64 Richard Ashcroft, 'Genetic information and "genetic identity"', p. 217.

Chapter 10   Moral Luck and Global Ethics

1 Williams, 'Moral luck', p. 24.
2 In addition to Williams's dismissal as a 'cop-out' of any other ending to the Pedro and Jim story than the two he presents, see also his essay 'Utilitarianism and moral self-indulgence'.
3 British Medical Association, *The Medical Profession and Human Rights*.
4 K. Cham et al., 'The impact of charging for insecticide', summarized in British Medical Association, *The Medical Profession and Human Rights*, p. 224.
5 M. Angell, 'The ethics of clinical research in the third world'; P. Aaby et al., 'Ethics of HIV trials'; P. Luria and S. M. Wolfe, 'Unethical trials of interventions to reduce perinatal transmission'; N. A. Halsey et al., 'Ethics and international research'.
6 See, for example, CIOMS in collaboration with WHO, *International Ethical Guidelines for Biomedical Research involving Human Subjects*; M. Clark et al., 'Ethical issues facing medical research in developing countries'.
7 Peter A. Sy, 'Rape research and research capitalism in Philippine bio-medicine'.
8 Solomon Benatar, 'Avoiding exploitation in clinical research' and 'Safeguarding participants in clinical trials'.
9 Salim S. Abdool Karim, 'The ethics of research in less developed countries'.
10 For example, the consultation exercise on ethics of research in developing countries undertaken in 2000–2001 by the Nuffield Council on Bioethics.
11 Bernard Williams, *Ethics and the Limits of Philosophy*, p. 195.
12 Ibid.
13 Ibid.
14 Ibid.

15   Ibid.
16   Bernard Williams, 'Persons, character and morality', p. 18.
17   MacIntyre, *Whose Justice? Which Rationality?*, p. 4. Formulating the content of ethical systems in terms of justice and rationality, as MacIntyre does, might itself be seen as the inheritance of the very Enlightenment project against which MacIntyre inveighs. Not every ethical or religious system would accept the connection between the two: limited human rationality needs to be transcended in order to enact the rule of divine justice on earth, in many religious systems.
18   Ibid., pp. 5–6.
19   Ronald Dworkin, 'Liberalism'.
20   MacIntyre, *Whose Justice? Which Rationality?*, p. 7.
21   For a coherent critique of value pluralism from the standpoint of a philosopher who has lived and worked in the developing world, where implementing health-promotion measures for women often runs up against the charge that traditional values are being overridden, see Sirkku Kristiina Hellsten, 'Multicultural issues in maternal-fetal medicine'.
22   MacIntyre, *Whose Justice? Which Rationality?*, p. 7.
23   Ibid., pp. 9–10.
24   Ibid., p. 10.
25   Ibid., p. 346.
26   Ibid., p. 353ff.
27   Ibid., p. 327.
28   Ibid., p. 334.
29   Marcia Baron, 'Kantian Ethics', p. 16.
30   MacIntyre, *Whose Justice? Which Rationality?*, p. 5.
31   O'Neill, *Towards Justice and Virtue*, p. 6.
32   Ibid., p. 16. O'Neill intends this criticism to apply particularly to John Rawls and Ronald Dworkin.
33   Ibid., p. 55, original emphasis.
34   Alan Gewirth, *Human Rights*; 'Rights and virtues'; 'Ethical universalism and particularism'.
35   O'Neill, *Towards Justice and Virtue*, p. 19.
36   Ibid., p. 53.
37   See, *inter alia*, the essays in Anthony McGrew (ed.), *The Transformation of Democracy*, and in David Held and Anthony McGrew (eds), *The Global Transformations Reader*.
38   O'Neill, *Towards Justice and Virtue*, p. 20.
39   Ibid., n. 31, pp. 28–9.
40   Ibid., p. 37.
41   Dickenson, *Property, Women and Politics*, especially chapter 1, 'Property, particularism and moral persons'.
42   O'Neill, *Towards Justice and Virtue*, p. 55.

43 The classic text of principlism in the United States is Tom L. Beauchamp and James F. Childress's *Principles of Biomedical Ethics*, although the tone of the 4th edition is less stringently autonomy-centred than that of its predecessors. The most long-standing and influential critic of the dominant emphasis on patient autonomy is probably Daniel Callahan: see, for example, his contribution to the colloquium 'Can the moral commons survive autonomy?'.

44 O'Neill, *Towards Justice and Virtue*, p. 58.

45 The Human Rights Act, which came into effect in 2000 as part of domestic English law following the incorporation of the European Convention on Human Rights, has the weakness of being such a catalogue, so that the precise rights to which it gives rise will become clear only with the development of case law.

46 A707/B735 (Prussian Academy pagination, in O'Neill's own translation), cited in O'Neill, *Towards Justice and Virtue*, p. 61.

47 O'Neill, *Towards Justice and Virtue*, pp. 62–3, original emphasis.

48 Martha C. Nussbaum, *Women and Human Development*, p. 5.

49 Ibid., original emphasis.

50 Ibid., e.g., p. 78; p. 80, n. 6.

51 See Dickenson, *Property, Women and Politics*, 'Introduction', for further substantiation of this claim.

52 Nussbaum, *Women and Human Development*, p. 74.

53 Ibid., p. 5. See also her argument on p. 83.

54 Ibid., p. 49.

55 Ibid., p. 77.

56 E.g., on p. 99.

57 Preamble to the Constitution of the Republic of South Africa Act no. 108 of 1996, cited in Ngwena and Engelbrecht, 'Health care professionals and conscientious objection to abortion in South Africa', p. 4.

58 Hoffmann *v.* South African Airways ([2000] (11) BCLR 1211, CC), at para 38, cited ibid.

59 Nussbaum, *Women and Human Development*, p. 83.

60 Ibid., p. 97.

61 E.g., Butler, *Subjects of Desire*, and Irigaray, *Ethique de la différence sexuelle, Sexes et parentés, Speculum of the Other Woman, Le temps de la différence*, and *This Sex Which is Not One*. For a more complete discussion of both writers, see chapter 6 of my *Property, Women and Politics*.

62 These categories are used by Kathy Ferguson in her book *The Man Question*, e.g., p. 14.

63 Ferguson, *The Man Question*, p. 5.

64 A similar position is taken by Susan Sherwin in *No Longer Patient*, chapter 2, distinguishing 'feminine' theories such as the ethics of care, which reinforce existing stereotypes about women's caring nature, from

truly 'feminist' theories, which are concerned primarily with the exploitation of women.

65   Margaret Whitford, *Luce Ingaray*, p. 83.
66   Among many examples, see Geetanjali Gangoli, 'The right to protection from sexual assault'; Haleh Afshar, 'Gendering the millennium'; Josefina Stubbs, 'Gender in development'; Kausar Khan, 'Justice and research in relation to women'; Nussbaum, *Women and Human Development*; and Sirkku Hellsten, 'Multicultural issues in maternal-fetal medicine'.
67   Iris Marion Young, *Justice and the Politics of Difference*, p. 105.
68   Ibid., p. 98.
69   Uma Narayan, *Dislocating Cultures*, p. 146, cited in Tong, 'Is a global bioethics both desirable and possible?'.
70   Susan Moller Okin, 'Feminism, women's human rights and cultural differences', p. 42.
71   Alison Jaggar, 'Toward a feminist conception of moral reasoning', p. 115.
72   Rosemarie Tong, 'Is a global bioethics both desirable and possible?', p. 24.
73   See, for example, Mary Mahowald, *Genes, Women, Equality*, chapter 1.
74   Susan Sherwin, 'Moral perception'.
75   Young, *Justice and the Politics of Difference*, p. 3.

Bibliography

Adshead, Gwen, and Dickenson, Donna, 'Why do doctors and nurses disagree?', in Donna Dickenson and Malcolm Johnson (eds) *Death, Dying and Bereavement* (London: Sage, 1993), pp. 161–8.

Advisory Committee on Genetic Testing, *Report on Genetic Testing for Late Onset Disorders* (London: Health Departments of the UK, 1998).

Afshar, Haleh, 'Gendering the millennium: globalising women', in Deborah Eade and Ernst Ligteringen (eds), *Debating Development* (Oxford: Oxfam UK, 2001), pp. 336–47.

Airedale NHS Trust *v.* Bland ([1993] 1 All ER 821).

Alderson, Priscilla, *Children's Consent to Surgery* (Buckingham: Open University Press, 1994).

—— *Choosing for Children* (Oxford: Oxford University Press, 1990).

Allain, Hervé, 'New drug therapies: how far can we stretch ethics? Country report on EBM in France', paper presented at the Maastricht Evibase workshop, 2 February 2001.

Alleback, P., Bolund, C., and Ringback, G., 'Increased suicide risk in cancer patients', *Journal of Clinical Epidemiology*, 42 (1989), pp. 611–16.

Allmark, Peter, 'Can there be an ethics of care?', *Journal of Medical Ethics*, 21 (1995), pp. 19–24.

Anderson, Elizabeth, 'Is women's labor a commodity?', in Anderson, *Value in Ethics and Economics* (Cambridge, MA: Harvard University Press, 1993), pp. 168–89; rev. in *Philosophy and Public Affairs*, 19 (1990), pp. 71–92.

Andre, Judith, 'Nagel, Williams and moral luck', *Analysis*, 43 (1983), pp. 202–7.

Andrews, Keith, Murphy, Lesley, Munday, Ros, and Littlewood, Clare, 'Misdiagnosis of the vegetative state: retrospective study in a rehabilitation unit', *British Medical Journal*, 313 (1996), pp. 13–16.

Anna J. *v.* Mark C. ([1991] 286 Cal. Rptr. 369).

Andrews, Lori B., 'Alternative modes of reproduction', in Sherrill Cohen and Nadine Taub (eds), *Reproductive Laws for the 1990s* (Clifton, NJ: Humana Press, 1989), pp. 380–8.

—— 'Surrogate motherhood: the challenge for feminists', in Larry Gostin (ed.), *Surrogate Motherhood: politics and privacy* (Bloomington: Indiana University Press, 1989), pp. 380–8.

Angell, Marcia, 'The ethics of clinical research in the third world', *New England Journal of Medicine*, 337 (1997), pp. 847–9.

Argyle, Michael, *The Psychology of Happiness* (London: Methuen, 1987).

Ashby, Michael, and Stoffell, Brian, 'Artificial hydration and alimentation at the end of life: a reply to Craig', *Journal of Medical Ethics*, 21 (1995), pp. 135–40.

Ashcroft, Richard, 'Genetic information and "genetic identity"', in Alison K. Thompson and Ruth F. Chadwick (eds), *Genetic Information* (New York: Kluwer Academic/Plenum Publishing, 1999), pp. 207–18.

—— 'Teaching for patient-centred ethics in medicine', paper presented at the 12th annual conference of the European Society for Philosophy of Medicine and Health Care, Marburg, Germany, 21 August 1998.

Baron, Marcia W., 'Kantian ethics', in Marcia W. Baron, Philip Pettit and Michael Slote, *Three Methods of Ethics* (Oxford: Blackwell, 1997), pp. 3–91.

Battin, Margaret P., 'Age rationing and the just distribution of health care: is there a duty to die?', *Ethics*, 97:2 (1987).

Bauer, Mark S., 'Bipolar disorders', in Allan Tasman, Jerald Kay and Jeffrey Lieberman (eds), *Psychiatry* (Philadelphia: W. B. Saunders, 1997), p. 969.

Beauchamp, Tom L., and Childress, James F., *Principles of Biomedical Ethics* (Oxford and New York: Oxford University Press, 2nd edn, 1983; 4th edn, 1994).

Benatar, Solomon, 'Avoiding exploitation in clinical research', *Cambridge Quarterly of Healthcare Ethics* (2000).

—— 'Safeguarding participants in clinical trials', *The Lancet*, 355 (2000), p. 2177.

Benhabib, Seyla, 'On Hegel, women and irony', in Mary Lyndon Shanley and Carole Pateman (eds), *Feminist Interpretations and Political Theory* (Cambridge: Polity, 1991), pp. 129–45.

Benner, Patricia, 'A dialogue between virtue ethics and care ethics', *Theoretical Medicine*, 18:1–2 (1997), pp. 47–61.

Bennett, Catherine, 'The baby incubators—yours for just £2 an hour', *The Guardian* (16 August 2001), section 2, p. 5.

Berg, M., 'Problemen en potenties van het protocol, de voorwaarden om protocollen positief in te zetten', *Medisch Contact*, 11 (1996), 366–70.

—— *Rationalizing Medical Work: decision support techniques and medical practices* (Maastricht: Rijksuniversiteit Limburg, 1995).

Bertelsen, A., 'A Danish twin study of manic-depressive disorders', in M. Schou and E. Stroemgren (eds), *Prevention and Treatment of Affective Disorders* (London: Academic Press, 1979).

Bewley, Susan, 'Restricting the freedom of pregnant women', in Donna L. Dickenson (ed.), *Ethical Issues in Maternal-Fetal Medicine* (Cambridge: Cambridge University Press, 2002), pp. 131–45.

Blum, Laurence, *Friendship, Altruism and Morality* (London: Routledge & Kegan Paul, 1980).

Bolam *v.* Friern Hospital Management Committee ([1957] 1 *Weekly Law Reports* 582).

Bolitho *v.* City and Hackney Health Authority ([1998] AC 232, HL).

Borger, Julian, 'All sides angry at Bush stem cell decision', *The Guardian* (11 August 2001), p. 17.

Bouchard, Thomas J. Jr., Lykken, David T., McGue, Matthew, Segal, N. L., and Tellegen, A., 'Sources of human psychological differences: the Minnesota study of twins reared apart', *Science*, 250 (12 October 1990), p. 223.

Boyd, Kenneth M., 'HIV infection: the ethics of anonymised testing and of testing pregnant women: Institute of Medical Ethics Working Party Report', *Journal of Medical Ethics*, 18 (1990), pp. 173–8.

Bradshaw, Ann, 'Yes! There is an ethics of care: an answer for Peter Allmark', *Journal of Medical Ethics*, 22 (1996), pp. 8–12.

Brahams, Diana, 'To be perfectly frank', *The Guardian* (25 June 1985).

Brandt, Richard B., *A Theory of the Good and the Right* (Oxford: Clarendon Press, 1979).

Bratty *v.* Attorney-General for Northern Ireland ([1963] AC 386, [1961] 3 All ER 523, HL).

Brazier, Margaret, 'Can you buy children?', *Child and Family Law Quarterly*, 11 (1998), pp. 345–54.

Brazier, Margaret, and Miola, Jose, 'Bye-bye *Bolam*: a medical litigation revolution?', *Medical Law Review*, 8:1 (2000), pp. 85–114.

British Medical Association, *Changing Conceptions of Motherhood: a report on surrogacy* (London: BMA, 1995).

—— *Children's Consent to Medical Treatment* (London: BMA, 2000).

—— *Human Genetics: choice and responsibility* (Oxford: Oxford University Press, 1998).

—— *The Medical Profession and Human Rights: handbook for a changing agenda* (London and New York: Zed Books, in association with the BMA, 2001).

Broad, C. D., 'The doctrine of consequences in ethics', in D. R. Cheney (ed.), *Broad's Critical Essays in Moral Philosophy* (London: Allen & Unwin, 1971), pp. 17–42.

Buckman, Robert, *I Don't Know What to Say: how to help and support someone who is dying* (London: Macmillan, 1988).

Butler, Judith, *Subjects of Desire: Hegelian reflections in twentieth-century France* (New York: Columbia University Press, 1987).

Calabresi, Guido, and Bobbitt, Philip, *Tragic Choices* (New York: W. W. Norton, 1978).

Callahan, Daniel, 'Can the moral commons survive autonomy?', *Hastings Center Report*, 26:6 (1996), pp. 41–7.

——*Setting Limits*: medical goals to an aging society (Washington, DC: Georgetown University Press, 1995).

——*The Troubled Dream of Life: living with mortality* (New York: Simon & Schuster, 1993).

Callahan, Joan C., 'Reconsidering parenthood: introduction', in Joan C. Callahan (ed.), *Reproduction, Ethics and the Law: feminist perspectives* (Bloomington: Indiana University Press, 1995), pp. 19–34.

Campbell, Alastair V., *Moderated Love: a theology of professional care* (London: SPCK, 1984).

Campbell, Alastair V., and Higgs, Roger, *In That Case: medical ethics in everyday practice* (London: Darton, Longman & Todd, 1982).

Canterbury *v.* Spence ([1972] 464 F 2d 772, DC).

Card, Claudia, *The Unnatural Lottery: character and moral luck* (Philadelphia: Temple University Press, 1996).

——'Women's voices and ethical ideals: must we mean what we say?' (review of Eva Feder Kittay and Diana T. Meyers (eds), *Women and Moral Theory*), *Ethics*, 97:2 (1992), pp. 374–86.

Chadwick, Ruth, 'Gene therapy and personal identity', in Gerhold K. Becker (ed.), *The Moral Status of Persons: perspectives on bioethics* (Amsterdam: Editions Rodopi, 1999), pp. 183–94.

Cham, K., et al., 'The impact of charging for insecticide on the Gambian National Bednet Programme', *Health Policy and Planning*, 12 (1997), pp. 240–7.

Charo, R. Alta, 'Bush's stem cell compromise: a few mirrors?', *Hastings Center Report*, 31:6 (2001), pp. 6–7.

Childress, James F., 'Who shall live when not all can live?', in Samuel Gorovitz et al. (eds), *Moral Problems in Medicine* (Englewood Cliffs, NJ: Prentice-Hall, 2nd edn, 1983), p. 642.

CIOMS [Council for International Organizations of Medical Sciences] and WHO [World Health Organization], *International Ethical Guidelines for Biomedical Research involving Human Subjects* (Geneva: CIOMS, 1993).

Clarke, Malcolm, Collinson, Andrew, Faal, Hannah, Gaye, Alieu, Jallow, Mariatou, Joof-Cole, Amie, McAdam, Keith, van der Loeff, Maarten Schim, Thomas, Vivat, and Whittle, Hilton (Gambia Government/MRC Joint Ethical Committee), 'Ethical issues facing medical research in developing countries', *The Lancet*, 351 (1998), pp. 286–7.

Clinical Genetics Society, 'The genetic testing of children: report of a working party', *Journal of Medical Genetics*, 31 (1994), pp. 785–97.

Clough, F., 'The validation of meaning in illness-treatment situations', in D. Hall and M. Stacey (eds), *Beyond Separation* (London: Routledge, 1979).

Cobbs *v.* Grant ([1972] 502 P2d 1).

Cochrane, Archie, *Effectiveness and Efficiency* (London: RSM Press, 1999); 2nd edn as *Effectiveness and Efficiency: random reflections on health services* (London: Nuffield Provincial Hospital Trust, 2001).

Cocks, Joan, *The Oppositional Imagination: feminism, critique and political theory* (London and New York: Routledge, 1989).

Cohen, L. Jonathan, *The Probable and the Provable* (Oxford: Clarendon Press).

Connolly, Kevin J., 'Genetics of behaviour', in Richard L. Gregory (ed.), *The Oxford Companion to the Mind* (Oxford: Oxford University Press, 1987), pp. 284–6.

Cooper, John M., review of Martha Nussbaum's *The Fragility of Goodness*, *Philosophical Review*, 97 (1988), pp. 543–63.

Coote, Anna, and Campbell, Beatrix, *Sweet Freedom: the struggle for women's liberation* (Oxford: Basil Blackwell, 1987).

Crabbe, Gill, 'The ultimate test', *Nursing Times*, 83:30 (1987).

Craig, Gillian, 'On withholding nutrition and hydration in the terminally ill: has palliative medicine gone too far?', in Donna Dickenson, Malcolm Johnson and Jeanne Samson Katz (eds), *Death, Dying and Bereavement* (London: Sage, 2nd edn, 2000), pp. 309–18.

Cruzan *v.* Director, Missouri Department of Health ([1990] 497 US 263).

Curry, Hazel, 'A dignified death', *The Guardian* (6 December 2001), section 2, p. 14.

Danis, M., Garrett, J., Harris, R., and Patrick, D. L., 'Stability of choices about life-sustaining treatments', *Annals of Internal Medicine*, 120 (1994), pp. 567–73.

Davey, Basiro, 'The nurse's dilemma: truth-telling or big white lies?', in Donna Dickenson and Malcolm Johnson (eds), *Death, Dying and Bereavement* (London: Sage, 1993), pp. 116–23.

Davidson, Donald, 'Belief and the basis of meaning', in D. Davidson, *Inquiries into Truth and Interpretation* (Oxford: Clarendon Press, 1984).

Davis, Glyn, Sullivan, Barbara, and Yeatman, Anna (eds), *The New Contractualism* (Melbourne: Macmillan Education Australia, 1997).

Department of Health, *Draft Arrangements for Inter-Agency Working for the Care and Protection of Severely Mentally Ill People* (London: Department of Health, 1994).

——*Surrogacy: Review for the UK Health Ministers of Current Arrangements for Payments and Regulation: consultation document and questionnaire* (London: Department of Health, 1997).

De Wert, Guido, Ter Meulen, Ruud, Tallachini, Mariachiara, and Mordacci, Roberto, *Ethics and Genetics Workbook* (London: TEMPE project, 2002);

246　Bibliography

pubd as *Genetics: teaching ethics, materials for practitioner education* (Oxford: Berghahn Books, 2002).

Dickenson, Donna, 'Are medical ethicists out of touch? Practitioner attitudes towards decisions at the end of life', *Journal of Medical Ethics*, 26 (2000), pp. 254–60.

—— 'Can children and young people consent to testing for adult-onset genetic disorders?', *British Medical Journal*, 318 (1999), pp. 1003–5

—— 'Can medical criteria settle priority-setting debates? The need for ethical analysis', *Health Care Analysis*, 7 (1999), pp. 131–7.

—— 'Commodification of human tissue: implications for feminist and development ethics', *Developing World Bioethics*, 2 (2002), 55–63.

—— 'Consent in children', *Current Opinion in Psychiatry*, 11 (1998), pp. 389–94.

—— 'Ethical issues in long-term psychiatric care', *Journal of Medical Ethics*, 23 (1997), pp. 300–4.

—— (ed.), *Ethical Issues in Maternal-Fetal Medicine* (Cambridge: Cambridge University Press, 2002).

—— 'Ethical issues in pre-cancer testing: the parallel with Huntington's Disease', in K. W. M. Fulford, Donna L. Dickenson and Thomas H. Murray (eds), *The Blackwell Reader in Healthcare Ethics and Human Values* (Oxford: Blackwell, 2002).

—— 'Is efficiency ethical? Resource issues in health care', in Brenda Almond (ed.), *Introducing Applied Ethics* (Oxford: Blackwell, 1995), pp. 229–46.

—— *Margaret Fuller: writing a woman's life* (Basingstoke: Macmillan, 1993).

—— *Moral Luck in Medical Ethics and Practical Politics* (Aldershot: Gower, 1991).

—— 'Nurse time as a scarce health care resource', in Geoffrey Hunt (ed.), *Ethical Issues in Nursing* (London: Routledge, 1994), pp. 207–17.

—— 'Property and women's alienation from their own reproductive labour', *Bioethics*, 15 (2001), pp. 205–17.

—— 'Property, particularism and moral persons', in Morwenna Griffiths and Margaret Whitford (eds), *Women Review Philosophy: new writing in philosophy* (Nottingham: University of Nottingham Press, 1996), pp. 45–68.

—— *Property, Women and Politics: subjects or objects?* (Cambridge: Polity, 1997).

—— 'Psychiatry, ethics and genetics', *Acta Geneticae Medicae et Gemellologiae*, 44: 2–3 (1995).

—— Review of Martha Nussbaum's *Women and Human Development*, *Monash Bioethics Review*, 20: 3 (2001), pp. 47–50.

—— 'The right to know and the right to privacy: confidentiality, HIV and health care professionals', *Nursing Ethics*, 1 (1994), pp. 111–118.

——'Who owns embryonic and fetal tissue?', in Donna L. Dickenson (ed.), *Ethical Issues in Maternal-Fetal Medicine* (Cambridge: Cambridge University Press, 2002), pp. 233–46.

Dickenson, Donna, and Fulford, K. W. M., *In Two Minds: a casebook of psychiatric ethics* (Oxford: Oxford University Press, 2000).

Dickenson, Donna, and Jones, David, 'True wishes: the philosophy and developmental psychology of children's informed consent', *Philosophy, Psychiatry and Psychology*, 2 (1995), pp. 287–304.

Dickenson, Donna, and Shah, Ajit, 'The *Bournewood* judgement: a way forward?', *Medicine, Science and Law*, 39 (1999), pp. 280–4.

——Letter, 'Bournewood: an indefensible gap in mental health law', *British Medical Journal*, 318 (1999), pp. 126–7.

Dickenson, Donna, and Viners, Paolo, 'Evidence-based medicine and quality of care', *Health Care Analysis*, 10 (3) (2002).

Discussion Group on Embryo Research [Canada], *Research on Human Embryos in Canada: final report* (Ottawa: Health Policy Division, 1995).

Dodds, Susan, and Jones, Karen, 'Surrogacy and autonomy', *Bioethics*, 3 (1989), pp. 1–17.

Donagan, Alan, 'Informed consent in theory and experimentation', *Journal of Medical Ethics*, 2 (1977), pp. 310–27.

Duff, R. A., *Intention, Agency and Criminal Liability* (Oxford: Blackwell, 1990).

Dunlop, R. J., Ellershaw, J. E., Baines, M. J., Sykes, N., and Saunders, C. M., 'On withholding nutrition and hydration in the terminally ill: has palliative medicine gone too far? A reply', *Journal of Medical Ethics*, 21 (1995), pp. 141–3.

Duxbury, Neil, *Random Justice* (Oxford: Oxford University Press, 1999).

Dworkin, Ronald, *Sovereign Virtue: the theory and practice of equality* (Cambridge, MA, and London: Harvard University Press, 2000).

——'Liberalism', in Stuart Hampshire (ed.), *Public and Private Morality* (Cambridge: Cambridge University Press, 1978), pp. 113–43.

Engelhardt, H. Tristram Jr., 'The crisis of virtue: arming for the cultural wars and Pellegrino at the lines', *Theoretical Medicine*, 18 (1997), pp. 165–72.

——*The Foundations of Bioethics* (Oxford and New York: Oxford University Press, 1986).

F. *v.* West Berkshire Health Authority ([1989] 2 All ER 545).

Faden, Ruth, et al., 'Disclosure of information to patients in medical care', *Medical Care*, 19 (1981), pp. 718–33.

Faulder, Carolyn, *Whose Body Is It? The troubling issue of informed consent* (London: Virago, 1985).

Feinberg, Joel, *Doing and Deserving* (Princeton, NJ: Princeton University Press, 1970).

Fenwick, P., 'Murdering while asleep', *British Medical Journal*, 293 (1986), p. 574.

Ferguson, Kathy E., *The Man Question: visions of subjectivity in feminist theory* (Berkeley, CA, and Oxford: University of California Press, 1983).

Field, David, *Nursing the Dying* (London: Tavistock/Routledge, 1989).

Field, Martha, 'Surrogate motherhood', in John Eekelaar and Petar Sarcevic (eds), *Parenthood in Modern Society: legal and social issues for the twenty-first century* (Dordrecht: Martinus Nijhoff, 1993), pp. 225–37.

Flew, Antony, *A Dictionary of Philosophy* (London: Pan/Macmillan, 1979).

Foucault, Michel, *Madness and Civilization: a history of insanity in the age of reason* (London: Tavistock, 1971).

Freeman, Michael, 'Does surrogacy have a future after Brazier?', *Medical Law Review*, 7 (1999), pp. 1–16.

Frenchay NHS Trust *v.* S ([1994] 2 All ER 403).

Freund, Paul A., 'Introduction: ethical aspects of experimentation with human subjects', *Daedalus* (1969), pp. 10–25.

Fries, James F., and Loftus, Elizabeth, series of letters in exchange with Ruth Barcan Marcus, Bruce Kuklick and Saevan Bercovich, *Science* (1979); repr. in Samuel Gorovitz et al. (eds), *Moral Problems in Medicine* (Englewood Cliffs, NJ: Prentice-Hall, 2nd edn, 1983), pp. 187–91.

Fulford, K. W. M., *Moral Theory and Medical Practice* (Cambridge: Cambridge University Press, 1989).

Fulford, K. W. M., Dickenson, Donna L., and Murray, Thomas H. (eds), *The Blackwell Reader in Healthcare Ethics and Human Values* (Oxford and New York: Blackwell, 2002).

Gangoli, Geetanjali, 'The right to protection from sexual assault: the Indian anti-rape campaign', in Deborah Eade (ed.), *Development and Rights* (Oxford: Oxfam UK, 1998), pp. 128–37.

Gatens, Moira, *Feminism and Philosophy: perspectives on difference and equality* (Cambridge: Polity, 1991).

—— 'Power, bodies and difference', in Michèle Barrett and Anne Phillips (eds), *Destabilizing Theory* (Cambridge: Polity, 1992), pp. 120–37.

Gauthier, Candace C., 'Teaching the virtues: justifications and recommendations', *Cambridge Quarterly of Healthcare Ethics*, 6 (1997), pp. 339–46.

General Medical Council, *Good Medical Practice* (London: GMC, 1995).

Gerrard, Eve, 'Palliative care and the ethics of resource allocation', in Donna Dickenson, Malcolm Johnson and Jeanne Samson Katz (eds), *Death, Dying and Bereavement* (London: Sage, 2nd edn, 2001), pp. 303–8.

Gewirth, Alan, *Human Rights: essays on justification and application* (Chicago: University of Chicago Press, 1982).

—— 'Rights and virtues', *Review of Metaphysics*, 38 (1985), pp. 739–62.

—— 'Ethical universalism and particularism', *Journal of Philosophy*, 85 (1988), pp. 283–302.

Gilbert, W., 'A vision of the grail', in Daniel J. Kevles and Leroy Hood (eds), *The Code of Codes: scientific and social issues in the human genome project* (Cambridge: Cambridge University Press, 1992).

Gillick *v.* W. Norfolk and Wisbech AHA ([1985] 3 All ER 402).

Gilligan, Carol, *In a Different Voice: psychological theory and women's development* (Cambridge, MA: Harvard University Press, 2nd edn, 1993).

Gillon, Raanan, *Philosophical Medical Ethics* (Chichester: John Wiley, 1986).

Glaser, B. G., and Strauss, A. L., *Awareness of Dying* (Chicago: Aldine, 1965).

Glover, Jonathan, *Causing Death and Saving Lives* (Harmondsworth: Penguin, 1977).

Gold, Richard E., *Body Parts: property and the ownership of human biological materials* (Washington, DC: Georgetown University Press, 1996).

Gowans, Christopher, *Innocence Lost* (Oxford: Oxford University Press, 1994).

Graves, Robert, *The Greek Myths* (London: Pantheon, 1960), vol. 2.

Green, R. M., 'Health care and justice in contract theory perspective', in R. M. Veatch and R. Branson (eds), *Ethics and Health Policy* (Cambridge, MA: Ballinger Publishing, 1976).

Greenspan, Patricia, *Practical Guilt* (Oxford: Oxford University Press, 1995).

Hall, Laura Lee (ed.), *Genetics and Mental Illness* (New York: Plenum, 1996).

Halsey, Neal A., Sommer, Alfred, Henderson, Donald A., and Black, Robert E., 'Ethics and international research', *British Medical Journal*, 315 (1997), pp. 965–6.

Hanford, Linda, 'Nursing and the concept of care: an appraisal of Noddings's theory', in Hunt, Geoffrey (ed.), *Ethical Issues in Nursing* (London: Routledge, 1994), pp. 181–97.

Harris, John, *Clones, Genes and Immortality* (Oxford and New York: Oxford University Press, 1999).

—— 'QALYfying the value of life', *Journal of Medical Ethics*, 13 (1987), pp. 117–23.

—— *The Value of Life* (London: Routledge, 1985).

—— *Violence and Responsibility* (London: Routledge & Kegan Paul, 1980).

Harrison, S., 'The politics of evidence-based medicine in the United Kingdom', *Policy and Politics*, 26 (1998), pp. 15–31.

Hartsock, Nancy C. M., *Money, Sex and Power: toward a feminist historical materialism* (Boston: Northeastern University Press, 1983).

Held, David, and McGrew, Anthony (eds), *The Global Transformations Reader* (Cambridge: Polity, 2001).

Hellsten, Sirkku Kristiina, 'Multicultural issues in maternal-fetal medicine', in Donna L. Dickensen (ed.), *Ethical Issues in Maternal-Fetal Medicine* (Cambridge: Cambridge University Press, 2002), pp. 39–60.

Hesselbrock, Victor M., 'The genetic epidemiology of alcoholism', in Henri Begleiter and Benjamin Kissin (eds), *The Genetics of Alcoholism* (New York: Oxford University Press, 1995), pp. 28–33.

Hinton, John, *Dying* (Harmondsworth: Penguin, 2nd edn, 1971).

Hirschmann, Nancy J., *Rethinking Obligation: a feminist method for political theory* (Ithaca, NY, and London: Cornell University Press, 1992).

Hope, Tony, 'Advance directives', *Journal of Medical Ethics*, 22 (1996), pp. 67–8.

—— 'Editorial: evidence-based medicine and ethics', *Journal of Medical Ethics*, 21 (1995), pp. 259–60.

Hurley, S. L., *Natural Reasons: personality and polity* (Oxford: Oxford University Press, 1989).

Hursthouse, Rosalind, 'Normative virtue ethics', in Roger Crisp (ed.), *How Should One Live? Essays on the virtues* (Oxford: Clarendon Press, 1996), pp. 19–36.

IHA [International Huntington Association] and WFN [World Federation of Neurology Research Group on Huntington's Chorea], 'Guidelines for the molecular genetics predictive test in Huntington's Disease', *Neurology*, 44 (1994), pp. 1533–6.

In re Jobes ([1987] 108 NJ 394).

In re Quinlan ([1976] 70 NJ 10).

In the Matter of Baby M ([1987] 217 NJ Supr. 313, affirmed in part and reversed in part [1988] 109 NJ 396.

Ingelfinger, Franz J., 'Informed (but uneducated) consent', *New England Journal of Medicine*, 287 (1972), pp. 465–6.

Irigaray, Luce, *Ethique de la différence sexuelle* (Paris: Editions de Minuit, 1984).

—— *Sexes et parentés* (Paris: Editions de Minuit, 1987).

—— *Speculum of the Other Woman*, tr. Gillian C. Gill (Ithaca, NY: Cornell University Press, 1985).

—— *Le temps de la différence: pour une revolution pacifique* (Paris: Livre de Poche 1989).

—— *This Sex Which is Not One*, tr. Catherine Porter with Caroline Burke (Ithaca, NY: Cornell University Press, 1985).

Jaggar, Alison M., 'Toward a feminist conception of moral reasoning', in James Sterba (ed.), *Moral and Social Justice* (Lanham, MD: Rowman & Littlefield, 1995).

Jaggar, Gill, 'Beyond essentialism and construction: subjectivity, corporeality and sexual difference', in Morwenna Griffiths and Margaret Whitford (eds), *Women Review Philosophy: new writing by women in philosophy* (Nottingham: Nottingham University Press, 1996), pp. 142–60.

Jamison, Kay Redfield, *Touched with Fire: manic-depressive illness and the artistic temperament* (New York: Free Press, 1993).

Jasanoff, S., *Science at the Bar: law, science and technology in America* (Cambridge, MA: Harvard University Press, 1995).

Jecker, Nancy S., 'Caring for "socially undesirable" patients', *Cambridge Quarterly of Healthcare Ethics*, 5 (1996), pp. 500–10.

Johnson, Alan G., *Pathways in Medical Ethics* (London: Edward Arnold, 1990).

Johnson *v.* Calvert ([1993] 851 P2d 776).

Jones, Kathleen B., *Compassionate Authority: democracy and the representation of women* (London: Routledge, 1993).

Kaasenbrood, J. A., 'Evidence based medicine en de dagelijkse psychiatrische praktijk', *Kwaliteit & Zorg*, 2 (1997), pp. 50–60.

Kaebnick, Gregory, 'Embryonic stem cells without embryos?', *Hastings Center Report*, 31: 6 (2001), p. 7.

Kahneman, D., and Varey, C., 'Notes on the psychology of utility', in J. Elster and J. E. Roemer (eds), *Interpersonal Comparisons of Well-Being* (Cambridge: Cambridge University Press, 1991), pp. 127–39.

Kant, Immanuel, *Critique of Practical Reason*, tr. Lewis White Beck (Indianapolis: Bobbs-Merrill, 1956).

——*Fundamental Principles of the Metaphysic of Morals (Grundlegung zur Metaphysik der Sitten)*, tr. Thomas K. Abbott (Indianapolis: Bobbs-Merrill, 1949).

——*Lectures on Ethics*, tr. Lewis White Beck (New York: Harper Torchbooks, 1963).

——*The Metaphysics of Morals*, tr. Mary J. Gregor as *The Doctrine of Virtue* (Philadelphia: University of Pennsylvania Press, 1964), part 2.

Karim, Salim S. Abdool, 'The ethics of research in less developed countries: the case of AIDS vaccine trials', paper delivered at the Fifth International Conference of the International Association of Bioethics, London, 21 September 2000.

Khan, Kausar, 'Justice and research in relation to women: it is not a matter of theory alone', paper delivered at the Fifth International Conference of the International Association of Bioethics, London, 21 September 2000.

Kirby, M. D., 'Informed consent: what does it mean?', *Journal of Medical Ethics*, 9 (1983), pp. 70–1.

Kleinig, John, *Ethical Issues in Psychosurgery* (London: George Allen & Unwin, 1985).

Kolata, Gina, 'Researchers find big risk of defect in cloning animals', *New York Times* (25 March 2001).

Komrad, Mark S., 'A defence of medical paternalism: maximising patients' autonomy', *Journal of Medical Ethics*, 9 (1983), pp. 38–44.

Kuhse, Helga, and Singer, Peter (eds), *Bioethics: an anthology* (Oxford: Blackwell, 1999).

Kyburg, Henry Jr., *Probability and the Logic of Rational Belief* (Middletown, CT: Wesleyan University Press, 1981).

Launis, Veikko, 'The concept of personal autonomy', in Michael Parker and Donna Dickenson, *The Cambridge Medical Ethics Workbook* (Cambridge: Cambridge University Press, 2001), pp. 280–3.

Law Commission, *Mental Incapacity* (London: HMSO, 1995), Law Comm. No. 231.

—— *Mentally Incapacitated Adults and Decision-Making: medical treatment and research* (London: HMSO, 1993), Law. Comm. No. 129.

Lee, Robert G., and Morgan, Derek, *Human Fertilisation and Embryology: regulating the reproductive revolution* (London: Blackstone Press, 2001).

Liechtenstein, Sarah, et al., 'Judged frequency of lethal events', *Journal of Experimental Psychology: human learning and memory*, 4 (1978), pp. 556–7.

Loewy, Erich H., 'Developing habits and knowing what habits to develop: a look at the role of virtue in ethics', *Cambridge Quarterly of Healthcare Ethics*, 6 (1997), pp. 347–55.

—— 'The uncertainty of certainty in clinical ethics', *Journal of Medical Humanities and Bioethics*, 8 (1987), pp. 26–33.

London, Alex J., and Knowles, Lori P., 'The Maltese conjoined twins – two views of their separation', *Hastings Center Report*, 31: 1 (2001), pp. 48–52.

Lord Chancellor's Department, *Making Decisions: the government's proposals for making decisions on behalf of mentally incapacitated adults* (London: Lord Chancellor's Department, 1999).

—— *Who Decides? Making decisions on behalf of mentally incapacitated adults* (London: Lord Chancellor's Department, 1997).

Louden, Robert, 'On some vices of virtue ethics', *American Philosophical Quarterly*, 21 (1984), pp. 227–36.

Luria, P., and Wolfe, S. M., 'Unethical trials of interventions to reduce perinatal transmission of the human immunodeficiency virus in developing countries', *New England Journal of Medicine*, 337 (1997), pp. 883–5.

Lynn, Joanne, 'Why I don't have a living will', *Law, Medicine and Health Care*, 19 (1991), pp. 101–14.

McCall Smith, R. A., 'When going to sleep is a crime', *The Times*, (17 October 1989), p. 36.

McCarthy, David, 'Rights, explanations and risks', *Ethics*, 107 (1997), pp. 205–24.

McDonagh, Eileen L., *Breaking the Abortion Deadlock: from choice to consent* (Oxford and New York: Oxford University Press, 1996).

McDowell, John, 'Virtue and reason', *The Monist*, 62 (1979), pp. 331–50.

McGrew, Anthony (ed.), *The Transformation of Democracy: globalization and territorial democracy* (Cambridge: Polity, 1997).

Mackie, John, *Ethics* (New York: Penguin Books, 1977).

MacIntyre, Alasdair, *After Virtue* (London: Duckworth, 1981).

—— *Whose Justice? Which Rationality?* (London: Duckworth, 1988).

MacKinnon, Catharine A., *Feminism Unmodified: discourses on life and law* (Cambridge, MA: Harvard University Press, 1987).

—— *Toward a Feminist Theory of the State* (Cambridge, MA: Harvard University Press, 1989).

Macklin, Ruth, 'Is there anything wrong with surrogate motherhood? An ethical analysis', in Larry Gostin (ed.), *Surrogate Motherhood: politics and privacy* (Bloomington: Indiana University Press, 1990), pp. 136–150.

McLean, Sheila A. M., 'Is there a legal threat to medicine? The case of Anthony Bland', second annual Centre for Applied Ethics public lecture, University of Wales College of Cardiff, 24 November 1992.

McNeil, Thomas F., 'Prebirth and postbirth influence on the relationship between creative ability and recorded mental illness', *Journal of Personality*, 38 (1971), pp. 391–406.

Maden, A., 'Risk assessment and management in psychiatry', *CPD Psychiatry*, 1 (1998), pp. 8–11.

Maher, G., 'Automatism and diabetes', *Law Quarterly Reports*, 99 (1983), p. 511.

Maher, G., et al., 'Diabetes mellitus and criminal responsibility', *Medicine, Social Science and Law*, 24 (1984), p. 95.

Mahoney, Joan, 'Adoption as a feminist alternative to reproductive technology', in Joan C. Callahan (ed.), *Reproduction, Ethics and the Law: feminist perspectives* (Bloomington: Indiana University Press, 1995), pp. 199–218.

—— 'An essay on surrogacy and feminist thought', in Larry Gostin (ed.), *Surrogate Motherhood: politics and privacy* (Bloomington: Indiana University Press, 1990), pp. 183–97.

Mahowald, Mary B., 'As if there were fetuses without women: a remedial essay', in Joan C. Callahan (ed.), *Reproduction, Ethics and the Law: feminist perspectives* (Bloomington: Indiana University Press, 1995), pp. 199–218.

—— 'The fewer the better? Ethical issues in multiple gestation', in Donna L. Dickenson (ed.), *Ethical Issues in Maternal-Fetal Medicine* (Cambridge: Cambridge University Press, 2001), pp. 243–55.

—— *Genes, Women, Equality* (Oxford and New York: Oxford University Press, 2000).

Mallia, Pierre, 'Letter: Maltese conjoined twins', *Hastings Center Report*, 31: 6 (2001), p. 4.

Malone, Caroline, Farthing, Linda, and Marce, Lorraine (eds), *The Memory Bird: survivors of sexual abuse* (London: Virago, 1996).

Marshall, Sandra, 'Whose child is it anyway?', in Derek Morgan and G. Douglas (eds), *Constituting Families* (Stuttgart: Franz Steiner, 1994).

Marx, Karl, *Grundrisse: foundations of the critique of political economy*, tr. Martin Nicolas (New York: Vintage Books, 1973).

Mason, J. K., 'The legal aspects and implications of risk assessment', *Medical Law Review*, 8 (2000), pp. 69–84.

Mason, J. K., and McCall Smith, R. A., *Law and Medical Ethics* (London: Butterworths, 3rd edn, 1991).

Medical Research Council, *Report of the MRC Working Group to Develop Operational and Ethical Guidelines for Collections of Human Tissue and Biological Samples for Use in Research*, Fourth Working Draft (London: MRC, 1999).

Mednick, S. A., Gabrielli, W. F., and Hutchings, B., 'Genetic influences in criminal convictions: evidence from an adopted cohort', *Science*, 224 (1984), pp. 891–3.

Meek, James, 'The brain gain', *The Guardian* (14 August 2001), section 2, p. 4.

Mele, Alfred R., *Autonomous Agents: from self-control to autonomy* (Oxford: Oxford University Press, 1995).

Mendlewicz, Julien, 'Genetics of depression and mania', in Anastasios Georgotas and Robert Canero (eds), *Depression and Mania* (New York: Elsevier, 1988), pp. 197–213.

Montgomery, Jonathan, *Health Care Law* (Oxford: Oxford University Press, 1997).

Moore, G. E., *Ethics* (London: Oxford University Press, 1912).

Moore *v.* Regents of the University of California ([1990] 51 Cal. 3d 120).

Morrison, Toni (ed.), *Race-ing Justice, En-Gendering Power* (New York: Pantheon, 1992).

Murdoch, Iris, *The Sovereignty of Good* (New York: Schocken Books, 1971).

Murray, Thomas, 'Attending to particulars', in Thomas H. Murray, Barbara A. Koenig and Judith Wilson Ross, 'Does clinical ethics distort the discipline?', *Hastings Center Report*, 26:6 (1996), pp. 28–34.

Nagel, Thomas, 'Moral luck', in *Mortal Questions* (Cambridge: Cambridge University Press, 1979).

—— *The View from Nowhere* (Oxford: Oxford University Press, 1986).

Narayan, Uma, *Dislocating Cultures: identities, traditions and third-world feminisms* (New York: Routledge, 1997).

Nelkin, Dorothy, and Lindee, M. Susan, *The DNA Mystique: the gene as a cultural icon* (New York: W. H. Freeman, 1995).

Nelson, Hilde Lindemann, and Nelson, James Lindemann, *The Patient in the Family* (London: Routledge, 1995).

Nesson, Charles, 'Reasonable doubt and permissible inference: the value of complexity', *Harvard Law Review*, 92 (1979), pp. 187–225.

Ngwena, Charles, and Engelbrecht, Michelle, 'Health care professionals and conscientious objection to abortion in South Africa: some legal and ethical responses', paper presented at the Second International Conference on Development Ethics, Tampa, Florida, February, 2001.

Novack, D. H., et al., 'Changes in physicians' attitudes toward telling the cancer patient', *Journal of the American Medical Association*, 241 (1979), pp. 879–900.

Nozick, Robert, *Anarchy, State and Utopia* (New York: Basic Books, 1974).

—— *The Nature of Rationality* (Princeton, NJ: Princeton University Press, 1993).

Nuffield Council on Bioethics, 'Consultation on behavioural genetics', (2001), <www.nuffieldfoundation.org/bioethics>.

—— *Mental Disorder and Genetics: the ethical context* (London: Nuffield Council on Bioethics, 1998).

Nussbaum, Martha C., *The Fragility of Goodness: luck and ethics in Greek tragedy and philosophy* (Cambridge: Cambridge University Press, 1986).

—— *Women and Human Development: the capabilities approach* (Cambridge: Cambridge University Press, 2000).

Oakley, Justin, 'A virtue ethics approach', in Michael Parker and Donna Dickenson, *The Cambridge Medical Ethics Workbook* (Cambridge: Cambridge University Press, 2001), pp. 296–304.

—— 'Altruistic surrogacy', *Bioethics*, 6 (1992), p. 269.

Oken, D., 'What to tell cancer patients', *Journal of the American Medical Association*, 175 (1961), p. 120.

Okin, Susan Moller, 'Feminism, women's human rights and cultural differences', *Hypatia*, 13: 2 (1998), pp. 32–52.

—— 'John Rawls: justice as fairness – for whom?', in Mary Lyndon Shanley and Carole Pateman (eds), *Feminist Interpretations and Political Theory* (Cambridge: Polity, 1991), pp. 181–98.

O'Neill, Onora, *Towards Justice and Virtue: a constructive account of practical reasoning* (Cambridge: Cambridge University Press, 1996).

Oppenheimer, Catherine, 'Ethics and psychogeriatrics', in Sidney Bloch and Paul Chodoff (eds), *Psychiatric Ethics* (Oxford: Oxford University Press, 2nd edn, 1991), pp. 365–90.

Oswald, I., and Evans, J., 'Serious violence while sleep walking', *British Journal of Psychiatry*, 147 (1985), p. 688.

Outka, G., 'Social justice and equal access to health care', *Journal of Religious Ethics*, 2 (1974), pp. 11–32.

Owen, C., Tennant, C., Levis, J., and Jones, M., 'Suicide and euthanasia: patient attitudes in the context of cancer', *Psycho-Oncology*, 1 (1992), pp. 79–88.

Parfit, Derek, *Reasons and Persons* (Oxford: Clarendon Press, 1984).

Parker, Michael, and Dickenson, Donna, *The Cambridge Medical Ethics Workbook* (Cambridge: Cambridge University Press, 2001).

Parker, Philip, 'Motivation of surrogate mothers: initial findings', *American Journal of Psychiatry*, 140 (1983), pp. 117–18.

Pateman, Carole, *The Sexual Contract* (Cambridge: Polity, 1988).

Pearce *v.* United Bristol Healthcare NHS Trust ([1999] PIQR 53).

Pellegrino, Edmund D., 'Toward a virtue-based normative ethics for the health professions', *Kennedy Institute of Ethics Journal*, 5 (1995), pp. 253–77.

Pellegrino, Edmund D., and Thomasma, David C., *The Virtues in Medical Practice* (New York: Oxford University Press, 1993).

Pelosi, Anthony J., and David, Anthony S., 'Ethical implications of the new genetics for psychiatry', *International Review of Psychiatry*, 1 (1989), pp. 315–20.

Phillips, Anne, *Engendering Democracy* (Cambridge: Polity, 1991).

Plato, *Protagoras*, in Edith Hamilton and Huntington Cairns (eds), *The Collected Dialogues of Plato* (New York: Bollingen Foundation/Pantheon Books, 1961), pp. 308–52.

Plomin, Robert, DeFries, John C., McClearn, Gerald E., and Rutter, Michael, *Behavioural Genetics* (New York: W. H. Freeman, 3rd edn, 1997), p. 228.

Price, D. P. T., 'Organ transplant initiatives: the twilight zone', *Journal of Medical Ethics*, 23 (1997), pp. 170–5.

Prior, A. N., 'The consequences of actions', *Proceedings of the Aristotelian Society*, 30 (1956), suppl.

Putnam, Daniel A., 'Virtue and the practice of modern medicine', *Journal of Medicine and Philosophy*, 13 (1988), pp. 433–43.

Quaid, Kimberley, Dinwiddie, Stephen H., Conneally, P. Michael, and Nurnberger, John N. Jr., 'Issues in genetic testing for susceptibility to alcoholism: lessons from Alzheimer's Disease and Huntington's Disease', *Alcoholism: clinical and experimental research*, 20 (1996), p. 1430.

R. *v.* Bailey ([1983] 2 All ER 503; [1983] 1 WLR 760, CA).

R. *v.* Cambridge Health Authority, ex parte B ([1995] 2 All ER 129, CA).

R. *v.* Quick ([1973] QB 910, [1973] 3 All ER 347, CA).

Radin, Margaret J., *Contested Commodities: the trouble with trade in sex, children, body parts and other things* (Cambridge, MA: Harvard University Press, 1996).

Ragone, Helena, *Surrogate Motherhood: conception in the heart* (Boulder, CO: Westview Press, 1994).

Rawls, John, *A Theory of Justice* (Cambridge, MA: Harvard University Press, 1971).

—— *Political Liberalism* (New York: Columbia University Press, 1996).

—— *The Law of Peoples* (Cambridge, MA: Harvard University Press, 1999).

Re an Adoption Application (Surrogacy) ([1987] 2 All ER 826).

Re C ([1994] 1 All ER 819).

Re E ([1993] 1 FLR 386, [1994] 2 FLR 1065).

Re MB (an adult: medical treatment) ([1997] 2 FCR 541).

Re T ([1992] 4 All ER 649).

Re W ([1992] 4 All ER 627).

Rescher, Nicholas, 'Moral luck', in Daniel Statman (ed.), *Moral Luck* (Albany: State University of New York Press, 1994), pp. 141–66.

Reznek, L., *The Philosophical Defence of Psychiatry* (London: Routledge, 1991).

Richards, Norvin, 'Luck and desert', in Daniel Statman (ed.), *Moral Luck* (Albany: State University of New York Press, 1994), pp. 167–80.

Robertson, David W., 'Ethical theory, ethnography, and differences between doctors and nurses in approaches to patient care', *Journal of Medical Ethics*, 22 (1996), pp. 292–9.

Robinson, George, and Merar, Avram, 'Informed consent: recall by patients tested postoperatively', in Samuel Gorovitz et al. (eds), *Moral Problems in Medicine* (Englewood Cliffs, NJ: Prentice-Hall, 2nd edn, 1983), pp. 279–84.

Roth, Loren H., Meisel, Alan, and Lidz, Charles W., 'Tests of competency to consent to treatment', *American Journal of Psychiatry*, 134 (1977), pp. 279–84.

Royal College of Paediatrics and Child Health, *Report of the Ethics Advisory Committee* (London: Royal College of Paediatrics and Child Health, 1997).

Russell, Bertrand, *Philosophical Essays* (London: Allen & Unwin, rev. edn, 1966).

Ryan, Christopher James, 'Betting your life: an argument against certain advance directives', in Donna Dickenson, Malcolm Johnson and Jeanne Samson Katz (eds), *Death, Dying and Bereavement* (London: Sage, 2nd edn, 2000), pp. 291–8.

Salgo *v.* Leland Stanford Jr. University Board of Trustees ([1957] 154 Cal. App. 2d 560, 317 P2d. 170).

Salsberry, Pamela J., 'Caring, virtue theory, and a foundation for nursing ethics', *Scholarly Inquiry for Nursing Practice*, 6 (1992), pp. 155–67.

Sanders, David, and Dukeminier, Jesse Jr., 'Medical advance and legal lag: hemodialysis and kidney transplantation', *UCLA Law Review*, 15 (1968), pp. 367–8.

Sard *v.* Hardy ([1977] 379 A.2d 1014, Maryland).

Savage, Wendy, 'Caesarean section: who chooses – the woman or her doctor?', in Donna L. Dickenson (ed.), *Ethical Issues in Maternal-Fetal Medicine* (Cambridge: Cambridge University Press, 2001), pp. 259–77.

Savulescu, Julian, 'Should we clone human beings? Cloning as a source of tissue for transplantation', *Journal of Medical Ethics*, 25 (1999), pp. 87–96.

Savulescu, Julian, and Dickenson, Donna, 'The time frame of preferences, dispositions, and the validity of advance directives for the mentally ill', *Philosophy, Psychiatry and Psychology*, 5 (1998), pp. 225–46.

Schloendorff *v.* Society of NY Hospitals ([1914] 105 NE 92).

Scruton, Roger, *Kant* (Oxford: Oxford University Press, 1982).

Seale, Clive, 'Demographic change and the experience of dying', in Donna Dickenson, Malcolm Johnson and Jeanne Samson Katz (eds), *Death, Dying and Bereavement* (London: Sage, 2nd edn, 2000), pp. 35–43.

Seale, Clive, and Cartwright, A., *The Year before Death* (Aldershot: Avebury, 1994).

Shah, Ajit, and Dickenson, Donna, 'The *Bournewood* case and its implications for health and social services', *Journal of the Royal Society of Medicine*, 91 (1998), pp. 349–51.

——'The capacity to make decisions in dementia: some contemporary issues', *International Journal of Geriatric Psychiatry*, 14 (1999), pp. 803–806.

Shanner, Laura, personal communication, 16 August 2001.

——*Embryonic Stem Cell Research: Canadian policy and ethical considerations*, report for Health Canada, Policy Division (31 March 2001).

Shaw, A. B., 'In defence of ageism', in Helga Kuhse and Peter Singer (eds), *Bioethics: an anthology* (Oxford: Blackwell, 1999), pp. 374–9.

Sherer, D. G., and Repucci, N. D., 'Adolescents' capacities to provide voluntary informed consent', *Law and Human Behaviour*, 12 (1988), pp. 123–41.

Sherlock, Richard, untitled contribution to symposium on consent, competence and electro-convulsive therapy, *Journal of Medical Ethics*, 9 (1983), pp. 141–3.

Sherwin, Susan, 'Moral perception: how global perspectives can inform and expand moral capacities in healthy ways', paper delivered at the Fifth International Conference of the International Association of Bioethics, London, September 2000.

——*No Longer Patient: feminist ethics and health care* (Philadelphia: Temple University Press, 1993).

Silver, R. L., and Wortman, C. B., 'Coping with undesirable life events', in J. Garberand and M. E. P. Speligman (eds), *Human Helplessness: theory and applications* (New York: Academic Press, 1980), pp. 279–340.

Slote, Michael, *From Morality to Virtue* (New York: Oxford University Press, 1992).

Smart, J. J. C., and Williams, Bernard, *Utilitarianism: for and against* (Cambridge: Cambridge University Press, 1973).

Smith *v.* Tunbridge Wells Health Authority ([1994] 5 Med. LR 334).

Smith, R., and Wynne, B. (eds), *Expert Evidence: interpreting science in the law* (London: Routledge, 1989).

Statman, Daniel (ed.), *Moral Luck* (Albany: State University of New York, 1994).

——'The time to punish and the problem of moral luck', *Journal of Applied Philosophy*, 14 (1997), pp. 129–36.

Stoop, A., Berg, M., and Dinant, G. J., 'Tussen afwijken en afwijzen van richtlijnen', *Huisarts en Wetenschap*, 1 (1998), pp. 5–9.

Stubbs, Josefina, 'Gender in development – a long haul, but we're getting there!', in Deborah Eade and Ernst Ligteringen (eds), *Debating Development* (Oxford: Oxfam UK, 2001), pp. 348–58.

Sy, Peter A., 'Rape research and research capitalism in Philippine biomedicine', paper presented at the Fifth International Association of Bioethics conference, London, 21 September 2000.

Szasz, Thomas, *The Myth of Mental Illness* (New York: Harper & Row, 1961).

Taylor, Charles, *Sources of the Self: the making of the modern identity* (Cambridge: Cambridge University Press, 1989).

Taylor, S. E., *Positive Illusions* (New York: Basic Books, 1989).

Teno, Joan M., et al., 'Do formal advance directives affect resuscitation decisions and the use of resources for seriously ill patients?', *Journal of Clinical Ethics*, 5 (1994), pp. 23–30.

Thomson, Judith Jarvis, 'A defense of abortion', *Philosophy and Public Affairs*, 1 (1971), pp. 47–66.

—— *The Realm of Rights* (Cambridge, MA: Harvard University Press, 1990).

—— *Rights, Restitution and Risk* (Cambridge, MA: Harvard University Press, 1986).

Tolstoy, Lev Nikolaievich, *Anna Karenina*, tr. Rosemary Edmonds (Baltimore: Penguin Books, 1954).

Tong, Rosemarie, 'Feminist perspectives and gestational motherhood: the search for a unified legal focus', in Joan C. Callahan (ed.), *Reproduction, Ethics and the Law* (Bloomington: Indiana University Press, 1995), pp. 55–79.

—— 'Is a global bioethics both desirable and possible?', paper delivered at the Fifth International Conference of the International Association of Bioethics conference, London, September 2000.

—— 'The overdue death of a feminist chameleon: taking a stand on surrogacy arrangements', *Journal of Social Philosophy*, 2:3 (1990), pp. 40–56.

Tsuang, Ming T., and Faraone, Stephen V., *The Genetics of Mood Disorders* (Baltimore: Johns Hopkins University Press, 1990).

US *v.* Holmes ([1841] 26 Fed. Cas. 360).

Vacco *v.* Quill ([1997] 521 US 793).

Vaillant, G., *Adaptation to Life* (Boston: Little Brown, 1977).

Van Hooft, Stan, 'Acting from the virtue of caring in nursing', *Nursing Ethics*, 6 (1999), pp. 189–201.

Van Rooy, Alison, 'Good news! You may be out of a job: reflections on the past and future 50 years for Northern NGOs', in Deborah Eade and Ernest Ligteringen (eds), *Debating Development: NGOs and the future* (Oxford: Oxfam Publishing, 2001), pp. 19–43.

Veatch, Robert M., *Death, Dying and the Biological Revolution* (New Haven, CT: Yale University Press, 1989).

—— 'The danger of virtue', *Journal of Medicine and Philosophy*, 13 (1988), pp. 445–6.

Veatch, Robert M., and Fry, Sara T., *Case Studies in Nursing Ethics* (Philadelphia: J. B. Lippincott, 1987).

Vineis, Paolo, 'Italy country report', European Commission Framework Programme 5 Evibase project meeting, Maastricht, Netherlands, 2 February 2001.

—— *The Tension between Ethics and Evidence-Based Medicine* (Turin: University of Turin and CPO-Piemonte, 2000).

Von Wright, G. H., *The Logical Problem of Induction* (Oxford: Blackwell, 1957).

Walker, Margaret Urban, 'Geographies of responsibility', *Hastings Center Report*, 27:1 (1997), pp. 38–44.

—— 'Moral luck and the virtues of impure agency', in Daniel Statman (ed.), *Moral Luck* (Albany: State University of New York Press, 1994), pp. 235–50.

Walker, Martin, 'Luck of the draw for MS drug', *The Guardian* (8 January 1994).

Wallace, L., 'Informed consent in elective surgery: the "therapeutic" value?', *Social Science and Medicine*, 22 (1986), pp. 29–33.

Washington et al. *v.* Glucksberg, ([1997] 521 US 702).

Weinman, J., 'Providing written information for patients: psychological considerations', *Journal of the Royal Society of Medicine*, 88 (1990), pp. 303–5.

White, Nicholas P., 'Rational self-sufficiency and Greek ethics', *Ethics*, 99 (1988), pp. 136–46.

White, R., Carr, P., and Lowe, N., *A Guide to the Children Act 1989* (London: Butterworths, 1990).

Whitford, Margaret, *Luce Irigaray: philosophy in the feminine* (London and New York: Routledge, 1991).

Wilcox, Mark A., 'Egg sharing: an NHS consultant's view', *Reproductive Biomedicine Online*, 3: 2 (2001), pp. 88–9.

Wilkes, Eric (ed.), *A Sourcebook in Terminal Care* (Sheffield: Sheffield Printing Unit, 1986).

Wilkinson *v.* Vesey ([1972] 295 A.2d 676).

Williams, Bernard, 'A critique of utilitarianism', in J. J. C. Smart and Bernard Williams, *Utilitarianism: for and against* (Cambridge: Cambridge University Press, 1973).

—— 'Ethical consistency', in Bernard Williams, *Problems of the Self* (Cambridge: Cambridge University Press, 1973), pp. 166–86.

—— *Ethics and the Limits of Philosophy* (London: Fontana/Collins, 1985).

—— 'Moral luck', in Bernard Williams, *Moral Luck* (Cambridge: Cambridge University Press, 1981), pp. 20–39.

—— 'Persons, character and morality', in Bernard Williams, *Moral Luck* (Cambridge: Cambridge University Press, 1981), pp. 1–19.

—— 'Postscript', in Daniel Statman, (ed.), *Moral Luck* (Albany: State University of New York, 1994), pp. 250–8.

—— 'The self and the future', in *Problems of the Self* (Cambridge: Cambridge University Press, 1973).

—— 'Utilitarianism and moral self-indulgence', in Bernard Williams, *Moral Luck* (Cambridge: Cambridge University Press, 1981), pp. 40–53.

Wilson, Jamie, and Borger, Julian, 'Surrogate twins find new parents', *The Guardian* (14 August 2001), p. 6.

Winslow, G. R., *Triage and Justice* (Berkeley, CA: University of California Press, 1982).

Young, Iris Marion, *Justice and the Politics of Difference* (Princeton, NJ: Princeton University Press, 1990).

Zimmerman, Michael J., 'Luck and moral responsibility', *Ethics*, 97 (1987), 374–86.

Zulueta, Paquita de, 'The ethics of anonymised HIV testing of pregnant women: a reappraisal', *Journal of Medical Ethics*, 26 (2000), pp. 16–21.

—— 'HIV in pregnancy: ethical issues in screening and therapeutic research', in Donna L. Dickenson (ed.), *Ethical Issues in Maternal-Fetal Medicine* (Cambridge: Cambridge University Press, 2001), pp. 61–85.

Index